"In A Queer Dharma, *Jacoby Ballard offers* on how to root the timeless truths of wisdom and compassion in a contemporary commitment to justice for all. He brilliantly weaves together powerful stories from his life journey with profound explorations of complex topics including forgiving what seems unforgivable, equanimity in the midst of oppression, and the colonization and commodification of yoga. The meditations and reflections blended throughout are clear and inspiring. This book is a nuanced, courageous, and compassionate gift for our individual and collective liberation."

—SEBENE SELASSIE, author of *You Belong*

"Through Jacoby Ballard's homage to their teachers, offering of the teachings they embody, and awareness that more teachings will come forth through them, A Queer Dharma *is the guide and medicine that we need at this time. Ballard offers powerful teachings about compassion, forgiveness, righteous rage, love, God, and knowing we have a place here and that it is our birthright to inhabit it.* A Queer Dharma *weaves in feminist, Black, and queer theory, creating a pathway for us to consider our identities and complexities and see ourselves as more expansive than our bodies. Ballard reminds us we are here on purpose and calls us into deep inquiry and action. Stories of their study and practice of dharma, Buddhism, and yoga, a beautiful love letter to queer and trans folks, call for us to heal our collective trauma and invite readers to dig deeper, transform and be better, to shift the culture of yoga and spiritual practice and beyond. This book is a blessing and should be received as such."*

—MICHELLE C. JOHNSON, author of *Skill in Action*

"What a gift A Queer Dharma *is to the world! Filled with deep wisdom and vulnerability, Jacoby Ballard shares radically courageous teachings and practices for transforming our lives and our communities. Whether you are a curious new practitioner, a spiritual activist committed to social justice values, or a seasoned practitioner or teacher seeking to grow and stretch on your path, this book is a tremendous offering for befriending yourself and others and developing practices for building Beloved Community in brave and collaborative ways. Deep bows of gratitude to Jacoby Ballard for this timely medicine for these times of shift in the world."*

—BRENDA SALGADO, author of *Real World Mindfulness for Beginners*

"A Queer Dharma *is for all people—queer or straight—and for anyone who has struggled with societal labels or identity in the world of yoga, meditation, or just in everyday life. Jacoby Ballard shares a unique point of view and their own experiences, which can help open the reader's eyes to the need for diversity, acceptance, and inclusion.*"

—SHARON SALZBERG, author of *Real Happiness* and *Real Change*

"*Only when we fully hear the voices and lived experiences of our trans, gender-queer, and nonbinary family can we move toward being a more whole and inclusive society. With great courage and humility, Jacoby Ballard explores timeless wisdom and practices that call forth the Buddha nature in each of us and invite us to embrace all beings in our tender, open hearts.*"

—TARA BRACH, author of *Radical Acceptance* and *Radical Compassion*

"*Jacoby Ballard has written a book that is both a fire under us calling us, in our own way, to be accountable to creating a just world and a salve offering a hopeful vision for the future. He skillfully weaves in the wisdom of his elders and contemporaries while sharing his personal journey of trauma and healing as a trans person, yoga and mindfulness teacher, and social justice activist. His unique experience situates him between the binaries, not just of gender but of justice and healing. Jacoby is a fierce guide with a huge heart.* A Queer Dharma *is for anyone and everyone interested in personal, interpersonal, and collective healing.*"

—HALA KHOURI, co-founder of Off the Mat, Into the World and author of *Peace from Anxiety*

"*Ballard's book brilliantly describes through teaching, personal story, and collective narrative how we, regardless of who we are, are everything—our identities, our suffering, our joys, our trauma, our achievements, how we heal, and how we harm. And because each of our 'everything' is indispensable to the whole, every one of us is so worthy, needed, and valued in this life together.*"

—LARRY YANG, author of *Awakening Together*

"Jacoby has written a book that does a beautiful job of weaving between the deep wisdom of Buddhist meditation practice and yoga practice while modeling an accountable relationship to a cultural practice that is not his own. His approach is respectful: what is it to bring a queer lens to the traditions, the cultures that have emerged around those traditions in the US, and then to share practices that support individual and collective liberation? It's a cautious thing to bring a contemporary lens—in this case, queerness—to a thousands-years-old tradition. Jacoby manages to hit the balance well so that the end point gives us something that feels respectful, aligned, and powerful. Mixing personal stories with the teachings of his teachers, Jacoby manages to both offer concrete suggestions and then also, when there is no clear answer, to not be afraid of the not knowing."

—SUSAN RAFFO, Healing Histories Project and Relationships Evolving Possibilities

"Deeply vulnerable and deeply moving, A Queer Dharma offers lessons from Ballard's personal journey to the heart of the dharma, bringing the whole body and loving the whole self. This book is for anyone who has a body and seeks to love courageously with an open heart."

—AUTUMN BROWN, host of How to Survive the End of the World

"In A Queer Dharma, Jacoby Ballard's journey of self-acceptance in a world that wants to deny the existence of queer/trans bodies is a revolutionary story of how the practice and teachings of the Buddha can transform suffering into liberation, both individually and collectively. This book serves the healing of many of us who belong to oppressed and marginalized groups as well as being a guidebook for those who seek to be better allies in creating greater access and belonging."

—LA SARMIENTO, board president and teacher, Insight Meditation Community of Washington

"*Perspectives on Buddhism, yoga, queer yoga, capitalism, anger, self-love, compassion, oppression, the breath, and much more fill the pages of this amazing book. In* A Queer Dharma, *Jacoby tells the story of a life filled with challenges, pain, and awakenings. An evocative work, this book shines a light on the difficulties inherent in expressing oneself as queer or transgender. By sharing Buddhism and yoga's ancient practices, Jacoby teaches us the importance of forgiveness, experiencing anger, and refusing to internalize hatred. As a Black woman, I know the pain caused by racism, sexism, and xenophobia. I stand alongside those finding their voice, as they become who they truly are.* A Queer Dharma *is an insightful and noble work. Thank you, Jacoby.*"

—MAYA BREUER, vice president of cross-cultural advancement, Yoga Alliance

"*A heartfelt offering that invites all of us to pause, reflect, and dive deeper. Jacoby provides thoughtful insights and practices to help lead us toward a more evolved, loving, and compassionate society.*"

—COBY KOZLOWSKI, author of *One Degree Revolution*

"*Jacoby addresses a foundational question of this decade: who gets left out of the modern yoga, mindfulness, spirituality, and wellness worlds, and how do we remedy that? This book is filled with fresh insight, vulnerability, and generosity of spirit. Highly recommended for practitioners of yoga and mindfulness, yoga teacher training and dharma center directors, somatic educators and therapists, and anyone engaged in building a world with more inclusivity, equity, and belonging.*"

—BO FORBES, psychologist, somatic educator, and author of *Yoga for Emotional Balance*

"*Through personal narratives, eclectic spiritual teachings, and mindful practices,* A Queer Dharma *offers up a practical and spiritual pathway that, if applied, can dismantle the oppressive practices, both within ourselves and within our world, that cause so much suffering and harm. This powerful guide is recommended for the student who wants to understand more about the intersection of spiritual practice and social justice. It's for the activist who needs tools for self-regulation and support. It's for nonbinary, queer, and/or trans folk or any marginalized person desiring a compassionate narrative of a lived experience that may mirror aspects of their* own. It's for the teacher, the ally, the family member. It's for those of us in the dominant, mainstream culture who want to challenge the limitations of our awareness, as well as our participation in the systems designed for inequality and hardship. It's for anyone who wants to live by the principle of Ahimsa—the commitment to not cause harm and disrupt it when we see it—but don't quite know how to do that mindfully. It's for everyone who wants to understand the complexities of the human experience and discover tools to help integrate truth, discharge emotions, and surrender to the Spirit within. If you want to understand the connection between spiritual practice and justice ... read this book. If you want to participate in creating a world that is compassionate, healed, and whole ... make this book your own, do the work, and put Jacoby's words into action in all aspects of your life."

—SEANE CORN, co-founder of Off the Mat, Into the World and author of *Revolution of the Soul*

"A Queer Dharma *is an offering for every heart that has been broken, every body that has survived violence, and every mind that has internalized false limitations. Like a balm, it soothes broken places and unidentified wounds, and through Ballard's exquisitely honest and tender pen, will fashion grace and deep healing from the fragmenting impact of the societies we are born into. From Ballard's tales and experiences as an educator, a Buddhist, an activist, and a yoga teacher, we are gifted with the timely and priceless exemplar of how to embody yoga and live one's dharma: by courageously embracing suffering, harnessing it skillfully and with care, and transforming it into a rare and active expression of profound love in an oft-unloving world."*

—CRYSTAL MCCREARY, yoga, mindfulness, and health educator and author of *Little Yogi Deck*

"In A Queer Dharma, *Jacoby Ballard transforms his painful past into powerful teachings using the magical alchemy of spiritual practice. Jacoby offers a message of healing and transformation through a contemporary perspective on yoga and meditation. The message is that peace is available for all of us, regardless of our background or life experience. I pray that all yoga and meditation teachers read this book!"*

—JIVANA HEYMAN, director of the Accessible Yoga Association and co-founder of the Accessible Yoga School

"A Queer Dharma *is a brilliant and important book with a profound message. With wit, humility, and keen discernment, Jacoby shares insights and wisdom gleaned from the lived experience of being 'othered.' Othering is a fundamental aspect of the socially constructed framework that the ancients call maya. Maya, the ancients say, covers us like a veil. Guided by the wisdom teachings of Buddhism and yoga, Jacoby offers us a glimpse into the possibility beyond the veil. Jacoby has given us a gift. I hope everyone reads this book."*

—R. NIKKI MYERS, founder of Y12SR: The Yoga of
12-Step Recovery

"A Queer Dharma *sits steadfastly on a compelling precipice between brave, bold conviction and humble heart-guided revelation. Full of eye-opening, unflinching personal experiences and learnings, Jacoby leads the reader by the hand through his own journey, which is at turns painful, uplifting, insightful, and captivating. The more I read, the more I found myself feeling how overdue a book like Jacoby's is. He offers crucial guidance without ever shaming or scolding the reader. Instead, you'll find yourself on your own journey of inquiry, right beside Jacoby—and a what a rich and rewarding journey it is for any wanting to undertake the path toward greater compassion."*

—JURIAN HUGHES, Kripalu yoga teacher and trainer

"The dharma is the moment when our collective will to heal, to grow, and to love well was given a new voice. That voice has now been informed by countless moments of practice across thousand of years. Jacoby Ballard added their voice to the dharma as a student, a teacher, and now as an author, offering us a thoughtful, honest, useful book that I believe will support each of us as we work to become the person we aspire to be. Einstein wrote that we believe ourselves to be separate from each other and that this sense of separation forms a mental prison each of us lives in. In doing the work and writing this book Jacoby has offered us a path toward connection."*

—ROLF GATES, teacher and author

"A Queer Dharma *takes us by the hand and walks us, step by loving step, through the process of turning the painful into the sacred, the hidden into the path. In his seminal work, Jacoby Ballard shares an unflinching view of the pain we've collectively inherited as queer, queer-adjacent and nonqueer people surrounding gender and all of the intersections that cross it. Part semi-autobiographical confession, part satsang, this field guide to tenderhearted yet fierce action gives us not only the terrain we must traverse if we wish for collective liberation, but the practices that can transform us along the way. A Queer Dharma streamlines many voices of wisdom, and so is for queer folks remembering their own power, allies pursuing an honest answer, and seekers of all experience who wish to walk more compassionately through this world."*

—JORDAN SMILEY, co-director of Courageous Yoga

"*'No mud, no lotus' is a popular Buddhist catchphrase. A Queer Dharma actualizes it and offers all of us—people of all colors, genders, orientations, and faiths—possibilities to imagine how we too can blossom like a lotus from the mud that life has dealt us. Through his own journey of finding wholeness in his body—despite the violence of gender and whiteness—Jacoby gently invites us to do the same. Jacoby is a queer seer of our times and this book is an invitation to heal for anyone who is ready and willing to join him on the journey."*

—ANU GUPTA, founder and CEO of BE MORE with Anu

"A Queer Dharma *is a deep, liberatory exhale. It is inclusion. It is vulnerability. It is grace. It is strength. It is humanness. It is profound wisdom that transcends words because it is truly an invitation to embody our wholeness and light amid the darkness. This compassionate, spiritual, and intersectional guide is a must read for every yoga instructor to understand the intersections of systemic oppression and injustice while simultaneously tending to our own wounds and care. It offers an invaluable window into understanding how integral it is to ensure all humans feel seen, valued, and affirmed—just as they are. I am completely moved by this work of art and by the reminder to ground ourselves in the power, practices, and community of vicarious resilience."*

—ZAHABIYAH YAMASAKI, author of *Trauma-Informed Yoga for Survivors of Sexual Assault*

"A Queer Dharma *is a first aid kit loaded with fuel for the soul and balm for the heart.*"

—KATHRYN BUDIG, author of *Aim True* and co-host of
Free Cookies

"*The time is NOW for this book. With intimacy and vulnerability, Jacoby invites us into the power of compassion and life-changing transformation. This book, their stories and reflections, will shape the way we offer yoga in our communities.*"

—TEJAL PATEL, yoga teacher, founder of Tejal Yoga and
abcdyogi, and co-host of the podcast *Yoga Is Dead*

A
QUEER
DHARMA

A QUEER DHARMA

YOGA AND MEDITATIONS FOR LIBERATION

JACOBY BALLARD

**FOREWORD BY
SUSANNA BARKATAKI**

North Atlantic Books
Berkeley, California

Published by

North Atlantic Books
Huichin, unceded Ohlone land
aka Berkeley, California

Cover art © gettyimages.com/molotovcoketail
Cover design by Jasmine Hromjak
Illustrations by Elvis Bakaitis
Book design by Happenstance Type-O-Rama

Printed in the United States of America

A Queer Dharma: Yoga and Meditations for Liberation is sponsored and published by North Atlantic Books, an educational nonprofit based in the unceded Ohlone land Huichin (aka Berkeley, California), that collaborates with partners to develop cross-cultural perspectives, nurture holistic views of art, science, the humanities, and healing, and seed personal and global transformation by publishing work on the relationship of body, spirit, and nature.

North Atlantic Books' publications are distributed to the US trade and internationally by Penguin Random House Publishers Services. For further information, visit our website at www.northatlanticbooks.com.

Library of Congress Cataloging-in-Publication Data

Names: Ballard, Jacoby, 1980– author.
Title: A queer dharma : your liberation bound with mine / Jacoby Ballard.
Description: Berkeley : North Atlantic Books, 2021. | Includes
    bibliographical references. | Summary: "Queer critique, queer practice:
    embodied teachings for healing from trauma and social injustice"—
    Provided by publisher.
Identifiers: LCCN 2021016581 (print) | LCCN 2021016582 (ebook) | ISBN
    9781623176518 (paperback) | ISBN 9781623176525 (epub)
Subjects: LCSH: Homosexuality—Religious aspects--Buddhism. |
    Toleration—Religious aspects—Buddhism. | Transgender people—Religious
    aspects—Buddhism.
Classification: LCC BQ4570.H65 B35 2021 (print) | LCC BQ4570.H65 (ebook)
    | DDC 294.3/44408664—dc23
LC record available at https://lccn.loc.gov/2021016581
LC ebook record available at https://lccn.loc.gov/2021016582

2 3 4 5 6 7 8 9 KPC 26 25 24 23 22

North Atlantic Books is committed to the protection of our environment. We print on recycled paper whenever possible and partner with printers who strive to use environmentally responsible practices.

I dedicate this book to queer brilliance and resilience, and to all social movements and activists over time and around the world.

Acknowledgments

I AM GRATEFUL to all of the freedom fighters—now and across history, around the world. My life is indebted to yours; I am because we are. You are my possibility models, my teachers, my comrades, my beloveds, my students.

Thank you to Third Root. I want to thank everyone who was involved with and kept alive Third Root Community Health Center in Brooklyn—everyone who has been a trial or temporary member-owner, all of the practitioners and teachers, people who have served on the advisory council, students and clients, and all those who have offered generative and scathing critiques. Third Root was a dream of mine and made me grow in ways I never would have asked for. Thank you Green Wayland-Llewellin for dreaming it up; for seeing cement floors, pastel walls, and fluorescent lights and imagining a healing community center and building a great crew. Thank you to Dara Silverman: without your support at Third Root's beginning, it would not have been born. I have incredible gratitude for the long-term co-owners I served with: Julia Bennett, John Halpin, Ji-Hye Choi, Romina Rodriguez-Crosta, Telesh Lopez, Stephen Switzer, Geleni Fontaine, Jomo Alakoye-Simmons, and Sherley Accimé. A deep bow to Emily Kramer, who matched my vision and big picture with her nitty-gritty and detailed fastidiousness at Third Root, who has co-taught seven Queer and Trans Yoga retreats with me, and who was the first to read an early version of this manuscript: your nuts and bolts keep us all from falling apart.

Thank you to my colleagues. I want to thank Seane Corn for believing in my leadership, wisdom, and critique, for helping me heal, for lifting me up, and for always having my back. Thank you to Hala Khouri for teaching about trauma grounded in justice politics and for modeling Beloved Community again and again. Thank you to Susanna Barkataki for writing the foreword to this book, being a social justice comrade in the yoga and Buddhist worlds, and for our deep, ongoing solidarity with and love for one another. Thank you to Crystal McCreary for chasing me down the halls of Kripalu, listening to me, grounding me, and allowing me to hold you too—the trust we have in one another runs deep. Thank you to Leslie Booker for drawing me in to so many of these relationships that I now rely on, and for the work you do to keep changemakers grounded and well. Thank you to Kate Johnson for modeling a depth of integrity that I aspire to, again and again. Thank you to La Sarmiento for making the dharma fun, light, and deeply meaningful and inviting me into the leadership team for the annual LGBTQ meditation retreat at the Garrison Institute. Thank you to comrades at Off the Mat, Into the World: Suzanne Sterling, Anita Akhavan, Teo Drake, Kerri Kelly, Chelsea Roff, Melody Moore, Carrington Razook Jackson, and Chelsea Jackson Roberts. I want to thank leaders involved with the Yoga Service Council over the years: Molly Lannon Kenny, Mark Lilly, Amina Naru, Pamela Stokes Eggleston, Bob Altman, Jennifer Cohen Harper, Nikki Myers, Michelle Cassandra Johnson, and Matthew Remski. Thank you to everyone involved in Bending Towards Justice: Lisa Garrett, Yashna Maya Padamsee, Meredith Gray, RW Alves, Karishma Kripalani, nisha ahuja, Faith Bynoe, Avi Rosentalis, Mimi Budnick, and Iris Jacobs—we were a little early, but knowing you all and your work continues to motivate me. Thank you to Jana Long and Maya Breuer for building the Black Yoga Teachers Alliance and welcoming my support of y'all. Thank you to Brenda Salgado for your friendship, alliance, and leadership in healing, Buddhism, and social justice. Thank you to Molly Kitchen for taking a risk and allowing me to co-lead your teacher training (twice!), for your important Consent Cards that are sent all over the world, for being a confidant and comrade in the realm of social justice and yoga, and for parenting alongside one another.

Thank you to my teachers and healers. Thank you to Lillian McMullin of Waterville, Maine, for allowing yoga to transform you and teaching it in a way that transformed your students. Jaya Devi Bhagavati at Kashi Atlanta, your leadership within and beyond queer community and your modeling of spiritual solidarity and skillfulness in holding space remain pillars for me. Thank you to Laura Booker for being a skillful therapist over the ups and downs of my life in Brooklyn. Thank you to Brian Liem for your queerness, for bringing the wholeness of your life into OM Yoga Center in Manhattan, and for being welcoming to every damn student. Thank you to Jurian Hughes for modeling growth and ever-growing skillfulness as a teacher and teacher trainer. Thank you to Larry Yang for your unflinching leadership, fearlessness, kindness, and integrity, even in denying my request to be your mentee. Thank you to Pascal Auclair for modeling anti-racism at the front of the room and questioning my attachment to activist identity at the back of the room.

Thank you to social justice movement organizations that continue to guide me: the Committee in Solidarity with the People of El Salvador (CISPES), Project South, Jews for Racial and Economic Justice, the Challenging Male Supremacy Project, the Buddhist Peace Fellowship, and all those involved in the Healing Practice Space at the 2010 US Social Forum in Detroit. Thank you to Anjali Taneja, Susan Raffo, and Cara Page for your initiative and leadership in the field now widely known as healing justice. Thank you to Burke Stansbury, Krista Lee Hanson, Sha Grogan-Brown, and Jesse Werthman for being an awesome team at CISPES and for rooting and growing me within an organization with a legacy. Thank you to Autumn Brown and adrienne maree brown for your facilitation prowess, vision, and keeping us all on the path of love. Thank you to RJ Maccani for your alliance, humility, and commitment to restorative and transformative justice. Thank you to my White Healing group on Monday nights: your kindness, questions, queerness, and decades of experience in and deep commitment to anti-racism give me courage, strength, and tools.

Thank you to my friends. To Elizabeth Parks, my longest-standing friend, for not giving up on judgy twenty-year-old me, for trusting me with the light and shadows of your life, and for your feedback on my chapter on forgiveness. Thank you to Emily Millay Haddad, the first one to voice that I should write a book: thank you for believing in this before I did. Thank you to Keshia Williams for refusing to allow me to turn my back on myself. Thank you to Tessa Hicks Peterson for being in this work and working out the tough moments of it together, for laughter, for integrity, and for perseverance. Thank you to Nathalie Fischer-Rodriguez for chasing me down at the Pride barbeque and insisting that we be friends—I thank all the gods that you knew we were kindred. Thank you to Sebene Selassie for the insightful texts and phone calls at the eleventh hour of this project. Thank you to LiZhen Wang for your boundless presence, long-standing commitment to justice and practice, and for always bringing a smile to my face.

Thank you to my students. Thank you to the Queer and Trans Yoga students at the NYC LGBT Center, in Brooklyn, Rochester, Easthampton, Salt Lake City, in retreats, and virtually: I write this book to honor you. Thank you to Meredith Gray for showing up and recruiting friends over the years to Queer and Trans Yoga. Thank you to Julie Kingery for your practice in and out of academia and for supporting my offering again and again. Thank you to Jena Duncan for asking all the hard questions and being transparent about your tussles with the teachings and continuing anyways. Thank you to Cody Derrick for all the work we've already done together and all that is in store for us. Thank you to the attendees of the annual LGBTQ retreat at the Garrison Institute: your practice grounds me when I'm untethered and encourages me when doubt arises. Thank you to all those I've mentored, trained, and taught here and there or consistently week to week, for trying on the teachings and allowing them to live through you.

Thank you to Gillian Hamel and the whole team at North Atlantic Books for valuing this book and honoring my work by publishing *A Queer Dharma*. My proposal was a last-ditch effort and what I thought was a long shot, and this is what I got for submitting it anyway. Thank you to Alex Kapitan for your copyediting prowess, for your attention to details, and for keeping each sentence and chapter aligned with my vision and commitments.

I want to thank my mom, who unknowingly instilled feminist and social justice values in me, who creates community and family out of friendships, and who continues to bravely tread through the thick and thin with me. Thank you for putting up with being "Jacoby's mom" over the years, for your consistency of showing up, and for the depths of your integrity (as annoying as it can be at times!).

I most importantly want to thank my beloved partner and utmost teacher, Lezlie Frye, who continually deepens my practice of kindness and integrity and expands my awareness of injustices and systems of oppression, their history, and possible futures. I am a better person for being your person, more steeped in love due to your love. Thank you for being home and making a home with me over and over again.

Finally, much love to the children in my life: my own Giuseppi Nova, as well as Valentino, Adé, Lulu, James, Cyprus, and those yet to be born. I endeavor to continue working toward a world that cherishes, protects, and respects each of you intrinsically and undeniably.

Contents

Part 2 | Queering Yoga

Foreword

YELLOW AND GREEN leaves burst free on branches freed from winter's grasp on a cool spring day in 2015 where I found myself at a retreat center in upstate New York. I was feeling completely out of place as one of the only people of color there and was wondering what I was even doing there in the first place.

"Hey friend, want to go on a walk?" Jacoby came up beside me and asked, with a smile that gently communicated that they had a sense of what I was going through and that they might feel some of it as well.

Jacoby had reached out to me in 2015 after I wrote "How to Decolonize Your Yoga Practice," a howl from my heart for yoga culture and loss in the West, as well as a vision for preserving the tradition. The article resonated for Jacoby and I found an email in my inbox asking to connect. I would later find out that this is classic Jacoby. They are a community builder, a connector, over time, space, and location. When they meet someone they reach out right away.

Despite being a bit wary of talking with an unknown white person without having any context or trust built, we got on the phone. Soon we were chatting it up about our passion for the dharma and yoga, discussing the various Buddhist retreats and yogic training we had experienced, and marveling over how we felt like family even though we were so different. Immediately the relationship felt profoundly transparent, honest, and intersectional. I let Jacoby know I had just been deeply betrayed by a new self-proclaimed white ally who had said something that cost me my job at my place of work. As the only woman of color in a leadership position there, that firing was a deep and painful loss, and not just personally—it also felt systemic. Jacoby immediately understood and said they were glad that I trusted them with my tenderness. They then shared their own story of betrayal at a place of work, around their own identity as trans. I was furious on their behalf at the systemic injustice involved, just as they were on my behalf.

As we walked and talked that cool spring day, we solidified what had begun as a cautiously optimistic relationship of connection across difference. Of recognizing that as a cisgender woman I would have advantages and be invited into places that Jacoby wouldn't as a trans person—and that as a white person Jacoby would be invited into various circles and opportunities that would exclude me as a South Asian woman, especially in yoga and dharma spaces.

We formed a tacit agreement to uplift each other. At first, most of the labor happened from Jacoby toward me, and helped ease my distrust of white allies, which itself has been immensely healing. Jacoby suggested that I serve on the board of a reputable yoga organization, and it was only because of Jacoby's recommendation that I got the position. They brought me into a consulting opportunity with another major yoga organization. Later I was able to bring them in to another consulting opportunity with another organization. We each platformed one another in trainings we led in various capacities—not only as specializing in trans education or cultural appropriation but as the full and incredible yoga and meditation practitioners we each are in our own right, both inclusive of and beyond our unique identities.

A lot of the leadership roles I now hold would not have ever happened, or been possible, without Jacoby opening these doors for me. For those who know me or my work, I want you to take that in. This is the potential of intersectional uplift. Jacoby is someone who walks through a door and brings others with them. *A Queer Dharma* brings us through many doors with them.

The compassion, love, and tenderness that Jacoby offered to me is the continual gift you will receive as you read this book. You'll also receive Jacoby's incisive and insightful clarity, cultivated through years of struggle and practice. Committed to social justice community and alternative institutions, Jacoby's writing is based on a lived praxis. With so much grace and care, Jacoby shares deep and personal stories that connect us to powerful universal truths.

Just like the flowering of the new shoots of green on bare trees, Jacoby brings life wherever they go. The openness to the magic of a queer identity, of dharma beyond binaries and limitations, is so vivid throughout Jacoby's life and work. There are so many moments of this liberatory healing throughout their book, such as in the chapter "Compassion: The Violence Stops with Me," where Jacoby says, "Working to heal my trauma with cisgender straight men and let men into my heart heals generations of trauma. This is not just my own trauma, but that of anyone who has been harmed, assaulted, or killed by a masculinity that manifests as power over others, control of others, unstated abuse of others." This chapter ends, as each one does, with a compassionate meditation to extend the wisdom we gain from Jacoby's experience into our own lives and practices.

Through this book Jacoby gives us tools to use for compassion for ourselves and others. Blending their Buddha dharma training and yogic experience, in this book Jacoby gives us a clear vision for the possibilities of a queer and inclusive yoga. "Queer is more than a sexual orientation; it is a political identity, and most people who are specifically queer-identified have a progressive, anti-oppressive politic about them." This intersectional, anti-oppressive wisdom is what Jacoby lives and shares and invites us into as they offer concrete practices for inclusion based on class, race, gender, culture, religion, sexual orientation, immigration, incarceration status, and all the other varied identities that humans might hold. As an organizer with decades of experience building alternative institutions, Jacoby gives us the gift of the vision of what yoga and dharma traditions can become as they explore "liberatory models" of yoga.

True to the transparent person I've known them to be, they also do not shy away from the hard conversations and go right for the heart of race and class oppressions, addressing cultural appropriation directly and with humility while offering clear and powerful practices folks can do to uplift those from the source culture. Some of these practices include humility, generosity and gratitude, and reparations, which Jacoby shares about from their own experiences and offers helpful suggestions for readers to continue their work.

I've always known Jacoby as someone I can go to with my deepest sufferings and my deepest joys, and they hold us with care in the chapter "We Are Fabulous: An Invitation into Joy." As someone who has experienced immense trauma and also deep healing through these sacred traditions, Jacoby is uniquely situated to offer us the wisdom of walking the path with us.

As a cisgender person, it is my responsibility (and yours too, if you are cisgender) to platform, uplift, and include trans and nonbinary teachers. But this responsibility is not simply one of obligation toward equity or inclusion. This is a responsibility to our future as one of brilliance, magic, and expansion; one where queerness can thrive. Jacoby provides this opportunity so lovingly and generously to us through this book. As they say, "One of my gifts is that I am situated in between places. Between binary genders and sexual orientations. Between social justice and healing practices. I pray that we each bring our own unique gifts, that we cherish the gifts others bring as well, and that we protect one another's dignity, belonging, and safety along the way."

I can't wait for you to join the celebration in *A Queer Dharma.* Jacoby invites us to this party—to yoga and dharma beyond barriers and boundaries, full of joy, compassion, embodiment, and absolutely fabulous, queer heart and soul.

This book is magic. And so are you. As you read it let it soothe your heart and fire up your soul, let it invoke your unique and expansive identities, and let's continue to liberate together.

With honor, love, and fire,

Susanna Barkataki

Author of Embrace Yoga's Roots

Introduction

MEDITATION SAVED MY life when I was a teenager. I was bullied for six years for being perceived as queer in my small mountain town in Colorado. I wasn't out as queer yet, even to myself, but I was taunted, physically harassed, teased, dismissed, and mentally and emotionally manipulated by peers who perceived something different and seized upon me. Another queer kid in our high school died by suicide in our freshman year; I could have been right alongside him had I not studied meditation at that time. Beginning meditation in high school taught me focus, revealed an inherent goodness in me regardless of what was happening around me or being said about me, and a spaciousness inside that could never be taken from me.

After graduating high school, I left. I went almost as far away within the continental US as I could, to a small liberal arts college in Maine. It was a good college, I would be challenged, I would get to begin again, yada yada, but most importantly and entirely unconsciously, it was getting me away from Carbondale, Colorado. In my sophomore year of college, I was required to take yoga; we needed to fulfill a wellness credit in order to graduate, and all my other options had expired. I learned a way of embodiment and living my life from seventy-year-old teacher Lillian McMullin, and I have continued to practice and find some incredible teachers and guides on my journey around the United States (including in Atlanta, Ithaca, Santa Fe, New York City, the Finger Lakes region of New York, western Massachusetts, and now Salt Lake City).

For so long, although deeply committed to my practice, I felt that my practice didn't fit. My politics and my body were unwelcome in yoga spaces, and my practice was met with disdain or judgment from fellow social justice workers. In many ways, I agreed with my social justice colleagues' critiques—and several of them are presented here in part 2 of this book. Yet still I was committed to the practice, for it had stewarded me through coming out as queer, my grandmother's death, coming out as trans, coming out as a survivor of childhood sexual abuse, and countless difficult interpersonal dynamics and heartbreaks. I had faith that the practice strengthened my social justice work, my mind, and my body.

My yoga and Buddhist paths are deeply intertwined, though I am quite aware of their differences. I explore Buddhism not as a religion, but as a practice—something to try on and repeat again and again, reducing suffering over time as the Buddha invited us to. Evolving in the same geographic space, yoga and Buddhism share many teachings, including most of the heart practices that I offer in part 1, which are found both in the Yoga Sutras of Patanjali and in Buddhist lineages. I largely practiced and studied Buddhism on my own until I met a swell of yoga colleagues in Brooklyn who were also Buddhists and, in some cases, training to be Buddhist teachers within the Insight tradition, a descendent of Theravada Buddhism arising out of Sri Lanka, Myanmar, Thailand, Cambodia, and Laos. These colleagues were largely queer women of color, and I followed them into the spaces where they practiced, and so was generally protected from many of the microaggressions that I experienced in yoga settings where I ventured solo. In over twenty years of study, practice, and teaching, the philosophies, skills, and sanghas that I have encountered have been vital to my survival, finding my work in the world, and the health of my friendships and professional relationships. I have learned yoga and dharma from loving people with quite different life experiences than me.

My queer and trans identities deeply influence my experience of yogic and Buddhist teachings, for I experience both my identity and the teachings as political. For me, identifying as queer is a political label rather than simply a personal identity. *Queer* conveys a politics and commitment not only around issues deemed as "LGBTQ issues," but also around deportation and immigration policies, mass incarceration, food justice, housing justice, climate change, and other issues concerning power and oppression. Being queer means being committed to anti-oppression, justice, and liberation, including how I express my sexuality and gender. I use the words *trans* and *genderqueer* to describe my gender identity, and I don't identify as a binary trans person—as a trans man. I use both *he/him* and *they/them* pronouns; I'm sometimes perceived as a man, sometimes as a butch woman, and sometimes as someone androgynous. I carried and birthed my child but did not nurse him. Not often seeing myself reflected in mainstream yoga and Buddhism led to my work in the world: creating space for underrepresented people, doing diversity, equity, and inclusion work within yogic and Buddhist institutions, and supporting social justice organizations and organizers to be grounded, resourced, and resilient.

In some ways, being pushed out of mainstream yoga shoved me right into the arms and hearts of my most beloved colleagues, who are now powerfully evolving yoga in the US: women of color, queer folks, and disabled and fat yogis. By mainstream yoga, I mean the colonized form of yoga on Turtle Island that emphasizes physical attainment over spiritual attributes, that is driven by the capitalist pursuit of profit, that is laced with white supremacy and cultural appropriation and resistant to calls for accountability and justice. I have had painful experiences of being called a "lady" in yoga classes early in my transition, when every such comment stung and stunted me for days. I was in a two-hundred-person class where everyone laughed when the teacher said that a particular posture was great for "pregnant people," leaving the door open for the possibility of pregnant men and nonbinary people—an idea that was clearly laughable to all of the students except me. In 2018 I was a pregnant fella, sometimes perceived as a man with a beer gut, attending regular yoga classes and adjusting my practice to care for my body and babe-to-be, not discussing my pregnancy with teachers who I knew couldn't hold my complexity. I was fired by a yogic institution in New York for being trans; I continued to practice while refusing to enter a yoga studio for the next five years. I needed to heal. I needed to strengthen. Through my tears, my running out of spaces in fury, and my rants at the covers of yoga magazines, I found my beloveds—yogis so brilliant, heartfelt, and courageous. I would not wish the racism, transphobia, misogyny, ableism, and fatphobia of mainstream yoga on anyone, including myself; my practice and the teachings held and guided me through those harmful moments. My practice is stronger, my network more robust, and my work more spacious because I have been through the wringer.

My task, then, is to hold the door open for and offer myself up to others, as well—queer and trans people of color, disabled people, fat folks, formerly incarcerated folks, and undocumented folks: people who are targeted by much more violent forms of oppression than me due to their intersecting identities marking them in multiple categories. I am so excited by so many trans people of color finding their work within yoga, and I vow to support them however I can, as well as show up as an accomplice to other yogis facing different forms of oppression within yoga. I continually grow and evolve my practices of compassionate listening, support, moving back, partnering with, and offering up.

I also must say that I found refuge in yogic and Buddhist teachings, teachings that come from South Asia, because of my whiteness. My parents and ancestors gave up their own spiritual traditions, teachings, and rituals in order to be assimilated into whiteness. That ancestral loss failed me in moments of great need and left me searching among other traditions. I am therefore grateful to all of the ancestors of these practices and their living descendants, for I might not be alive today were it not for their generosity in sharing the teachings. As I write in the section on gratitude in the chapter on joy, when we are truly grateful for something or someone, we have a duty to reciprocate, steward, accompany, and support.

This book is a queer approach to the practices of yoga and Buddhism, exploring the teachings, critiquing mainstream yoga culture, and providing some examples of liberatory practices, both within ourselves and within organizations. My queer community has incredibly insightful and clear critiques (of yoga, Buddhism, pop culture anything, really), beautiful tender hearts caring for and fully showing up with the power of their presence and attention for themselves and others in our chosen families (when a baby is born, at funerals, at graduations, at organizations' ten-year anniversary celebrations, and more), and innovators and visionaries who are making old models of social movements obsolete, growing our influence, and winning not just policies but the hearts of many. I cite teachings and wisdom by social justice leaders and visionaries alongside that of yogis and Buddhist teachers—they are all my sangha, my mentors, my heroes, and my colleagues, so if you are approaching this book from the yoga or dharma side of things, there may be unfamiliar reference points and explorations. If that is the case, I invite you to read slowly, absorb, and reflect, cultivating curiosity and respect. If you are approaching this text from the social justice side of things, I invite your vulnerability through my own and your contemplations of how these practices might ground, evolve, and expand our movements and organizations, whether they are familiar or not within your own ancestry and spiritual practices.

This book is for my queer and trans community and siblings, to see some of your own experiences reflected in these pages. This book is for straight and cisgender people to learn about how yoga practice is experienced and expressed through one queer individual, with some different stories, reference points, and musings than you may be familiar with. This book is for fitness fanatics who pooh-pooh the spiritual dimensions of these practices. This book is for mental health workers who may not necessarily consider the body, or who may suggest yoga to a queer client without knowing the potential harm you may be sending them to. This book is for white yogis who either don't understand why cultural appropriation is a problem or drop the practice entirely, afraid to be one of the "bad white people" who practice yoga or Buddhism. This is for my beloveds and colleagues of color: an acknowledgement of harm and my complicity, a prayer for a world of equity, and a public commitment to steadfastly continue the work of racial justice. This is for those new to social justice movement work, hesitant to join, terrified of scathing critiques or being shunned in your not knowing. This is for my fellow social justice workers who need spaces and teachings to guide and hold your weary body/heart/mind. This is for all the martyrs out there, who keep on keeping on until something breaks—your partnership, your body, your resilience. This is for my queer comrades who are on the front lines of social change through art, philanthropy, theater, writing, scholarship, dance, and beyond. This is for the apolitical tenderqueer, inviting you out of your shell and validating your vulnerability. This is for those healing from trauma through practice and those healing the sources of trauma through movement work. This is for the healers holding important, necessary, vital space for bodies, hearts, and minds, for you to be held too, so that you can continue. This is for my colleagues in the yoga service and yoga and social justice fields, teaching in prisons and schools, in homeless shelters and on the US–Mexico border, adding my voice to your own and inviting those of you who haven't written to courageously share as I do here how the practices live in you—the world is in need of your wisdom and insight. This is for all the students, those practicing from within violent institutions and those who will never see the inside of those buildings, those comfortable practicing in studios and meditation halls and those who refuse to practice in a studio or meditation hall for your own well-being. This is for the elders who have been grappling with, navigating, and exploring these teachings for many decades, and this is for the young ones, including and beyond my own beloved Giuseppi Nova, who inherit the work we have done and the beautiful bodies of practice and communities of belonging that we have created, as well as our missteps and failures.

Part 1

QUEER DHARMA

MY LIFE EXPERIENCES have led me to my dharma—my life's work, and my offering to the world. The Brahma Vihara practices that I discuss have become my dharma: my duty, my path, and the only way through.

Dharma comes from the root word *dhri-*, which means "to be in alignment with the cosmic law," "to make whole," "duty," and "righteous action." Dharma has two different translations. In Buddhist traditions that are written in Pali, it means "the truth" or "teaching." In yogic traditions that are written in Sanskrit, it means "duty" or "calling." In this book, I call upon both translations. In this first part, I explore dharma as teachings of truth, and also as practices to be in alignment with all other beings, the earth, our ancestors, thereby carving a skillful, compassionate, and courageous path for our descendants.

In this first part I offer teachings with which I have grappled, struggled, challenged my teachers, danced with, and been stumped by. The Brahma Viharas are translated as "the dwelling places of the sacred" or "the heart practices"; they are found in many Buddhist lineages and also within the Yoga Sutras of Patanjali, and include the practices of lovingkindness, compassion, sympathetic joy, and equanimity. I also explore teachings around anger, letting go, and forgiveness, as they often arise while exploring the formal set of Brahma Viharas. These are also the teachings that I have come to live by. The teachings that I offer invite our own exploration and practice—just because they have reduced suffering for millions of humans before you or me doesn't guarantee that they will work for you or me! I offer to you how I have worked with them, include formal meditation instructions in each chapter, and invite you to integrate the teachings into the living of your life. Before I dive into the teachings, I'd like to introduce some of my teachers, whose teachings I work with in each chapter.

Swami Jaya Devi Sati Bhagavati is the founder of Kashi Atlanta and was one of the first teachers to cherish me, support me, and deeply challenge and push my practice. Her ashram was down the street from my apartment and she happened to be leading a two-hundred-hour teacher training at the time, her first. I had been teaching for two or three years already, without training. Jaya Devi has never let me off the hook; she has grown with me, has expressed wariness and guidance when I've been about to take a wrong turn, and has evolved to deeply support Black communities and teachers in Atlanta. In her arms I have come out as trans and mourned my grandmother's death. She is fierce, kind, clear, and models integrity.

Larry Yang is a gay Chinese American Buddhist teacher who I have sat with three or four times, and who has supported me individually over the years. I have had the honor to teach yoga at two LGBTQ meditation retreats he led with La Sarmiento and Madeline Klyne at the Garrison Institute in New York. Larry retired in 2018 after cultivating social justice in the Insight Buddhist lineage for years, including leading retreats for LGBTQ folks and people of color and pushing for the mentorship, training, and uplift of teachers of color. The dharma talks that Larry has given at the retreats I've attended with him are among the most pivotal teachings I've received, offering a depth of practice that supports social justice in our world.

Madeline Klyne is a white lesbian Insight teacher who trained alongside Larry in the Insight tradition, a founder of South Shore Insight, and a main teacher at the Cambridge Insight Meditation Center. She has been a lead teacher for each of the LGBTQ meditation retreats at the Garrison Institute, and I have been privileged to get to know and teach alongside her. Maddy is a consistent ally to communities of color and trans communities, ever growing, and has held space through big political moments such as the 2016 and 2020 elections. I consider her both a teacher and a friend on the path.

Seane Corn is a bridge between corporate and mainstream yoga communities and social justice yoga communities and has worked to make social justice and equity work more relevant and irresistible within mainstream yoga, while always supporting those at the margins. Ten years ago, I would have never imagined Seane would become one of my greatest teachers; she is among the most internationally recognized of yoga teachers, and she is kind, introspective, embodies integrity, and is always expanding her commitment to social justice. Seane has taught me how to remain committed and connected to the humanity of the most difficult people—for me, the most privileged. Seane opens doors and steps aside in the consistent and dedicated way that any ally to any community knows how to do. She listens, and out of her awareness and deep presence she remembers your name and where you're from, even if your interaction with her lasted only thirty seconds. I asked Seane to be a mentor to me and she gracefully declined, asking that we mentor one another instead.

Gina Sharpe is the founder of New York Insight Meditation Center, and a multiracial Jamaican and Chinese Buddhist teacher. I have never had the honor of sitting with Gina, but I know her teachings through friends who are her students as well as her writing, interviews, and dharma talks. She shares stories of being "the only one" in many retreats, and the loneliness and deepening of her practice in those experiences, which I really share. She and Larry Yang together have been a force for racial justice within the Insight Buddhist lineage.

Laverne Cox is the trans possibility model that I waited so long for! Both she and Leslie Feinberg are trans folks who live and breathe justice, unafraid to call out and call in and act and speak in solidarity with oppressed people. I've never met Laverne, but I long to. I know she has a meditation practice, and I don't think she considers herself a teacher; I consider her a teacher because of how fiercely committed she is to love and justice, how she loves on trans people, queer folks, and communities of color, and how she uses her spotlight to benefit others.

Some of my teachers are also healing justice, food justice, restorative justice, solidarity, racial justice, prison abolition, and transformative justice movements. I have worked within these movements and continue to study and learn from them. In these movements I've learned to discern what love is and what love is not, as Seane Corn puts it. I began my activism in 1998 through the anti-globalization movement against the World Trade Organization, International Monetary Fund, World Bank, Free Trade Area of the Americas, and the North American Free Trade Agreement. This led me into environmental justice, food justice, solidarity, and racial justice. Coming out as queer and trans naturally drew me into movements, networks, and organizations led by queer and trans folks, particularly queer and trans people of color building campaigns around local and national policies that impact our daily lives.

Too often, social justice and spiritual practice are seen as separate or even at odds with one another. Around 2006, there was a powerful call to understand healing as a form of social justice, which was disseminated through the 2007 and 2010 US Social Forums and their Healing Justice Practice Spaces, which I am grateful to have been a part of in 2010. Individual and collective healing is now recognized as imperative among some of the most inspiring and visionary social justice organizations and leaders in the country. Mainstream yoga and white Western Buddhist spaces have been slower to open up to social justice, but it is increasingly relevant and important since the 2020 Freedom Summer of racial justice uprisings in more than four hundred US towns and cities after the murders of George Floyd, Breonna Taylor, Ahmaud Arbery, and Tony McDade. In waves, yogis wake up to social justice as yoga—after Occupy Wall Street, amid the advent of the Black Lives Matter movement, in the wake of the 2016 election. There remains resistance and plenty of work to be done, and I am grateful to all of my colleagues in that work. We are many and ever-growing.

In some ways, I've learned what my work is by delving into what my work is not. I worked with the Committee in Solidarity with the People of El Salvador (CISPES) for two years, which led me to found Third Root Community Health Center in Brooklyn. I learned so much from the Salvadoran social movement and the longevity of CISPES solidarity activists, as well as the organization's evolution to be led by Salvadoran Americans as more and more Salvadorans immigrated to the US due to the harsh impact of neoliberal trade policies. As important as CISPES is, it wasn't my work.

I recognize that as a white masculine-identified person, I am protected from so many of the injustices and travesties that my siblings who are people of color and/or femme regularly experience; part of my responsibility in that recognition is a commitment to solidarity, acting as an accomplice, and leveraging my privilege. In the pages that follow, I offer stories from my path and the struggles and openings that I have had with each teaching, with the hopes that it will help others along the path of awakening and love, liberation, and freedom—or at least help clear some brush along the way.

ACCEPTANCE AND
LETTING GO

God doesn't make mistakes.
—SWAMI JAYA DEVI BHAGAVATI

LIVING AS QUEER, gender nonconforming, and trans people in the world is difficult—we are blessed by our bodies but don't always realize it, nor does society around us. Swami Jaya Devi would often say, "God doesn't make mistakes," and as I was initially coming out as trans I thought, "Yes, well, God did—I don't want this body that doesn't resonate with who I am inside; that was a mistake." At that time, in 2004, I was at the beginning of coming out as trans and I was confused, angry, and depressed. That state of being is a reasonable response to a transphobic world where gender dysphoria is considered a mental illness by the *Diagnostic and Statistical Manual of Mental Disorders* and where media portrayals of trans lives remain largely limited and reinforce the gender binary or feature tragic deaths of trans characters. As I came out as trans, I couldn't see beyond the horizon and I was incredibly impatient. Wells of anger and grief emerged as well—grief from childhood trauma, rage at my ancestors, fear about climate change, exhaustion from a society prioritizing profit over people, and a well of sadness at the impact of systems of oppression in my queer community.

"God doesn't make mistakes" is an important teaching for all of us targeted by systems of oppression. Many different social movements have done this embracing, from "Black Is Beautiful" to reclaiming the words *crip* or *queer*. We do this cultural work in our world, and we must attend to our hearts and minds as well. Shanesha Brooks-Tatum has said, "Black women's self-care is also subversive because to take care of ourselves means that we disrupt societal and political paradigms that say that Black women are disposable, unvalued. Indeed, people and things that aren't cared for are considered expendable. So when we don't take care of ourselves, we are affirming the social order that says [B]lack women are disposable."[1] Audre Lorde said, "Caring for myself is not self-indulgence, it is self-preservation, and that is an act of political warfare."[2] The women of the Combahee River Collective foresaw just that when they said, "If Black women were free, it would mean that everyone else would have to be free, since our freedom would necessitate the destruction of all systems of oppression."[3] I bow to these Black women and so many others who have not only led the way for the Black folks and other people of color who followed in their path, but also for their wisdom, courage, and vision that created room for my own life. When we work for the liberation of those most targeted and marginalized, the rest of us get freedom in the process.

"God doesn't make mistakes" goes beyond reclaiming and loving ourselves. It is also about accepting reality as it is, rather than how we would like it to be. If we can recognize the reality of right now, and bring the fullness of our experience (with all of our privileges and oppressions) into our awareness, then we can create the possibility of liberation in the next moment. With full awareness of life's ten thousand joys and ten thousand sorrows, we can change what comes next, the next moment, the next generation. We can learn to soften, to open up, to forgive this moment, so that the space and attention thereby created ensures that no further harm will be done.

I moved to New York City in 2005 because I had come out as trans and needed community. It was an unlikely and unforeseen move: I grew up in a rural town in the Rocky Mountains. I went to college in Maine and spent most of my days in the woods and on farms. I majored in environmental policy and conducted my thesis on the then-forthcoming USDA organic certification requirements. In my first year out as trans, I lived in social justice communities that were ignorant about gender identity, where queer cisgender women struggled with the idea of their friends and lovers transitioning. It was an irresistible move to New York City: a trans friend had moved to New York the previous year and was involved with a vast queer and trans community, a job I was qualified for was open at the natural food store where my friend worked, and a room in his apartment was available. I needed to be around other trans and genderqueer people for my own survival. What I needed, when I needed it most, appeared. God doesn't make mistakes.

I moved to New York and lived there for nine years. I met some of my closest friends there who are passionate about justice and community building and involved in some of the most innovative justice work in the country. I founded a worker-owned cooperative health center in Brooklyn during the 2008 economic crash. I met my life partner there. My journey as a trans person has opened me up to love and justice work in a way that couldn't be otherwise: it has made me vulnerable; it has meant that I face hate and misunderstanding. This body, this identity, and the world as it is right now create the possibility for my work *and* my liberation, which involves struggle, facing sorrow, and the hard creative work of possibility. In my twenties, as I came out, I was frustrated that others weren't doing or hadn't already completed the work at the intersection of social justice and healing. In hindsight, this frustration was insecurity, grief, fear, disbelief, and overwhelm: was I up for all this?

"God doesn't make mistakes" is a personal spiritual inquiry, not an assessment of an individual or our world. Like so many teachings, this is a teaching to take on personally, one that should not be prescribed by someone else, which would be paternalistic, demonstrate a lack of willingness to attend to the pain in others' lives, or be used as an excuse for injustice. This teaching allows me to approach life like waves that I am surfing, rather than as a battle that I am waging. It was offered by Jaya Devi, and I chose to take it on. If I believe that God doesn't make mistakes, that I am given these circumstances as an opportunity to grow, then it creates more spaciousness from which to approach different life circumstances. This teaching of "God doesn't make mistakes" invites us out of the victim mentality, to reclaim this moment, this day, in recognition of our trauma and the wisdom and compassion that can grow out of it. This teaching invites us to take on full responsibility for this moment—circumstances may be difficult, and even amid that, freedom is possible.

If I can have the space and practice to approach the heights of the waves and my own glory with detached appreciation (the practice of *mudita*), and to approach the strength and power of the ocean with patient compassion, knowing that this will also change (a phrase I have tattooed on my forearm), then I can maintain an equanimity that fosters my own happiness. If I approach it like a battle, I lose out on the opportunity for gratitude and appreciation, the opportunity to be generous with what I have because I am constantly clamoring for more, believing that I have not been given enough or was shortchanged or misunderstood.

Madeline Klyne asks, "What do you need to make room for, learn, or let go of in order to make room for the possibility of inner freedom right now?" The practice of mindfulness is a full commitment to each and every moment, an awareness in every moment that can lead to justice. How do we practice mindfulness in a way that enables us to "not add a single further drop of suffering to a world that already hurts so much," as Larry Yang encourages us? Can we live and practice in a way that allows room for mistakes and repair?

This teaching does not excuse or dismiss ingrained patterns of injustice or internalized oppression. I want to be careful not to use spiritual wisdom to justify hatred in the world. I am not saying that injustice is right or that I approve of it. I am talking about where we place our attention: if we place attention on everything that is wrong, disturbing, or deeply sad, over and over again in a daily way, how does that impact our capacity to thrive and envision? On the other hand, if we don't pay attention to all of the injustice in the world, and don't modify our own thoughts, words, and actions with the intention of not adding a single further drop of suffering, then we are not present with the world around us; we are living in a fantasy. We need balance. We need both.

"God doesn't make mistakes" creates the possibility of freedom. Embedded in this teaching is the notion that I am being cared for by the divine, no matter what. It takes the edge off of what I could see as a harsh reality and allows me to have a "don't know mind" about what may come next, as well as gratitude for my life, for all of the amazing changemakers that

I have the opportunity to live this life with, and for the gracious earth. If I wasn't exactly who I am—someone who struggles with my sarcastic family, someone who was fired for being trans, someone who grew up adjacent to the wealthiest county in the state, someone who lost my dad at age six, someone whose first boyfriend died by suicide, someone who is a second-generation incest survivor, and someone who has survived all of the other difficult circumstances that I have experienced—if all of this was different, I would not experience the depth of compassion and love that I do. My heart might not be as open or compassionate as it has grown to be as a result of everything that I have lived through. I can live with resentment, an attitude of "why me," or I can live with gratitude for the understanding and commitment to justice that my very life has entrusted me with. I was given a lot to hold, and if I can consider the possibility that this is because my soul is up for holding all of this enormity, then I can soften and trust myself, the divine, and the world around me. The teaching "God does not make mistakes" then points toward "why *not* me?"

"God does not make mistakes" invites us into an understanding that God also did not make mistakes with anyone else. It allows me the possibility of love for others—even homophobes, people who instigate wars, white supremacists and conspiracy theorists, and leaders of corporations that displace people from their traditional lands through mining or pipeline projects. This is a huge area of growth—learning to love unconditionally includes loving oppressors, with the understanding that "hurt people hurt people," a common Buddhist adage. Anyone creating war on the outside also has a war on the inside. I am not condoning or excusing any of this behavior but rather refusing to throw anyone away.

Oppressed people have a unique opportunity to teach the world about love. There is a story of Tibetan monks walking down a road and one asks the other, "Have you forgiven your captors yet?" The other says, "No, never!" Then the first monk says, "Well, then, they still have you in prison, don't they?"[4] If I replicate the behavior of someone who tells me that I am wrong for being queer or that I have a mental disorder for being trans by calling them crazy or saying that they are wrong or bad, I participate in separation and harm as well. I can only offer love to someone else once I am offering it to myself. If I can learn to see the pain of someone who harasses me on the subway, then I can connect with their humanity, rather than separating from them because of their words or punches.

The notion of "God does not make mistakes" necessitates some letting go, a letting go of that ideal reality and how I wish the world was right now. In the service of my own liberation, I need to accept this moment as it is rather than how I might like it to be and release my anticipation of both violence and freedom, to allow this moment to be what it is and learn from it.

PRACTICE: LETTING GO MEDITATION

Find a comfortable seat where you can pay attention and be present. Begin by paying attention to your exhale for a few minutes. This exhale is a letting go that has been present every breath of your life. You know how to let go.

Begin to consider something in your life that you have been holding on to. Allow yourself to feel that holding, clinging, grasping. Notice how that feels in your body. Imagine the future of this clinging—ten to twenty years from now how is your life, still holding on, still wrapped around this way of being, still clinging to a relationship being a certain way or to a more concrete identification with your work? Begin to consider what you might feel like, who you might be, if you were able to let that go. How would you carry yourself? How would you speak? How would you relate to others?

Now, as if sitting down to tea with what you are holding on to, begin to gently say, "I am letting you go." Repeat this on each breath, noticing what emotions or sensations arise. Continue to offer this for some time until it feels like the grasping has released. Then just allow yourself to sit with that spaciousness, of having released. If it arises again, as if it's knocking on your door, turn toward it again and offer, "I have let you go. I have let you go."

To close, let go of the words and just sit with your breath once again. Feel your body, allow thoughts to float through your mind, notice what kind of emotions emerge. You might close with a bow, as if bowing to the thing you were grasping for, as if a great teacher of the timeless lesson of letting go.

ANGER AND SUSTAINABILITY

The world won't stop being transphobic, misogynist, or homophobic: how do I continue to encounter that in a way that does me the least harm?

—SEANE CORN

IN A TRAINING of more than sixty people, we were all asked the question in small groups, "What breaks your heart?" I answered with a shaky voice, "All that my community endures and inflicts again on itself." I was thinking about drama in my community, the struggles over politics and love, incarceration, abuse when the systems designed to "help" often perpetuate more harm, the harassment we endure for dressing how we do or holding hands with a lover. I was thinking about unemployment rates among trans people. I was thinking about homicides and suicides of queer and trans people and how routinely such news arrives in my news feed, inbox, or voicemail.

Seane Corn reflected to me in this moment that I hold so much for my students and want to protect them from going through what I have gone through. She noticed some martyr qualities and told me that this way of being is unsustainable. She told me that not only can I not hold all of this for my vast community, but that it's not healthy to even try. As we spoke with sixty onlookers, she helped me uncover the rage in my belly and burning at my temples, my chin jutted back, my voice shut off, holding it all in. My body demonstrated not knowing how to safely express anger at injustice and fear of the grief underneath the rage.

Seane asked me how I can let this rage out, and asked if I would like to scream. Being a generally quiet and soft-spoken guy, I reluctantly agreed, and then breathed into my belly and let out a loud, guttural roar that I didn't think I was capable of. Seane asked me to do it two more times, and subsequently instructed me to go up on my roof in Brooklyn and yell as a yogic practice, in order to let out the tension and free myself from holding it all.

This lesson was a long time coming for me; I built my home with walls of anger for about a decade. Through my experience in social justice, part of my role and identity in being progressive and taking leadership is to be angry at injustice everywhere. I took up residence there, righteous, pointing fingers at family, friends, politicians, and corporations who were doing harm to people and the planet. I felt I would be irresponsible or unaware of the important issues at hand if I were not angry, if I were not looking for more injustices to align my life against. I had a bumper sticker on my car in college that said, "If you're not angry then you're not paying attention," which is a phrase that I *lived* during a decade of social justice work, up to that moment with Seane. Fueling my anger was judgment—judgment of any behavior or language that wasn't "on point," not understanding or forgiving ignorance despite the fact that I had also been and remain ignorant of many particular sufferings.

Underneath anger is a broken heart. Once the anger has cooled, the task is to be present to the tender broken heart—the hurt, betrayal, disappointment, and grief. Lama Rod Owens says, "The work to turn our attention back to the woundedness is this really intense, profound path of transformation, which doesn't feel as good as just responding to the anger, because the energy of anger makes us feel powerful. Some of us, particularly if we're coming from positions and communities where we feel marginalized or erased, use that anger to feel powerful, to feel valid."[1] There is this vulnerability of being with the pain, and many of us have learned that vulnerability is a risk, potentially threatening our lives. The practice of being with pain is very tender. If we don't tend to the hurt, we cannot transform it into something else. It will seep out. We work with the resistance to being with our pain, and we work with pain itself.

Sometimes anger is not a choice, as we need this fire for our survival. Anger is important: it tells us that something is wrong; it is a human emotion that we can't remove or exorcise from our human experience. We need anger to ignite our social justice movements, but it needs to be balanced with self-care practices, with compassion and love for one another, and perhaps even with compassion and love for our "enemy." We need to fuel our movements with emotions besides anger.

I imagined that the goal of activism was to eliminate all harm, and that activists fail if we replicate harm. Perhaps eliminating harm remains the goal. There are innumerable causes for my anger: the privatization and pollution of water; the state-sanctioned violence against Black, Brown, fat, queer, feminine, and disabled bodies; the US material support of harmful governments around the world; the homicide and suicide of queer and trans folks; the high incidence of childhood sexual abuse; the vast wealth disparity within the US and the history of that wealth disparity (stolen land, stolen bodies, stolen labor). I honor my anger. Our world doesn't have to be this way; collectively and individually, we could be making kinder choices with more integrity, placing people and planet before profit. My anger is a dreamer—it knows that another world is possible. My anger is a toddler—it wants that world *right now!*

The activist circles I was part of in my twenties had no patience for the transformation of one's politics and practice. Thich Nhat Hanh teaches about anger being a ball of fire we intend to hurl at someone else, but in the process our own hands get burned. We need concrete practices to be with and move through anger, or we will burn our hands, our households, our communities, our potential bridges and alliances. What I have learned through yoga is that this anger is a fire that can eat me alive if I stay there. Anger is useful and motivating, and its passion is important, but we must uncover the immense grief, disappointment, and impulse to protect what is most sacred that lies beneath it and transform its fire into a sustainable commitment to justice fueled by love.

Working with Anger and Grief

It is very important to recognize and work with anger, for you don't want to heal over the wound without healing the wound itself. I am recalling here the medicinal qualities of calendula, which is so good at healing skin that it can even help skin heal over an infection, thereby sealing the infection inside the skin. We need to get curious about the wound, tend to it with presence and tenderness, and trust the healing process.

Anger is important and wise. We need to feel its seething fires and righteous indignation. We need to be present to our anger, like a screaming young child trying to tell us something. What does your anger have to tell you? What is it bringing to your attention about what is important to you? What is wrong? Anger deserves attention and requires a patient and enduring witness. And we don't want to get stuck there.

We turn toward pain with compassion practices. We seek witness and guidance from comrades who have shared experiences, embody courageous presence, and offer mentorship. We take strength in all those who have turned toward their pain and recycled it into commitment, kindness, and integrity, setting them on our altar as a reminder of why we are bothering to do this. We turn toward anger because the only way is through, as Yoga of 12-Step Recovery teacher Nikki Myers says.

Discharging Anger's Energy

We need to release anger's energy through a discharge practice, something I learned from my colleague Hala Khouri. There are innumerable discharge practices around the world, including singing, drumming, dancing, stomping, and screaming. This is so important! We see animals discharge all the time as a transition practice. I witnessed therapeutic horses working with trans kids at a camp where I was a counselor. When the child or adult was finished with the horse, the horse's caretaker would take the horse for a short walk, and in that process inevitably the horse would flutter its lips and shake its skin. Discharge is natural and normal for our animal friends.

A well-known example of discharge is often shown in Somatic Experiencing training (a therapy developed by Peter Levine that connects trauma responses to the body), where an opossum gets attacked by a wolf. The opossum only has one tool—to play dead. It can't outrun the wolf and it can't effectively fight the wolf. So it rolls over and plays dead, becomes stiff, closes its eyes, emits an odor conveying to the wolf that it is not live prey. The wolf is not interested in dead prey, so it walks away. Once safe, the opossum runs its little legs, while still upside down. Then it flips onto its feet, shakes its whole body, walks away, and gets on with its day. The opossum was discharging the fight-or-flight energy by "running away." Its nervous system then got to feel successful—it ran, it survived, it shook it off, and it continued living its opossum life.

Many of us have a discharge practice but don't recognize it as such. Going to the batting cages, boxing, and sex can all be discharge practices— they allow for moving energy and letting go with grunts and heavy exhales. When we recognize our go-to discharge practice, we can engage it with intention, especially when the going gets tough and there is potent energy to release. My discharge practices are *pranayama* (yogic breath practices), running, yelling on mountaintops, and push-ups. We can anticipate when we might need to move energy—like my friend dropping her child off with her ex, the child's co-parent. Ooh those exchanges can have some energy, especially if the breakup was recent! My friend wisely plans to go to the batting cages afterward to let the tension out.

The importance of discharge is that if you don't release anger's potent, fiery energy, then it is going to come out in all the wrong places—when a partner puts a dish in the wrong spot, when a child creates a mess, when the dog won't cooperate (yes, all examples from my life right now). In those small upsets lies all the anger one has pent up within—what is released is not just about the dish, the mess, the dog! Hala says "when it's hysterical, it's historical." It's not just about that moment if the reaction outsizes the moment.

Discharge allows you to retain the wisdom of the anger that tells you that something is wrong and communicate in a grounded way. Once the clenched belly, tight lips, or heat in the body has been released or worked through, your tone and body language will more effectively deliver the message. We receive a person's tone and body language far before the words, so we will notice angry tones or angry body language if that energy is present. We will likely shut down or go into protective mode.

The anger isn't wrong or bad; it's natural and human! Anger's energy can supersede the important, wise message. You are protecting the wisdom of the anger by discharging anger's energy. You are ensuring a more skillful delivery and better chances of a fruitful conversation about a necessary shift or an uncommunicated need.

Relating to Harm Skillfully in Community

How can I wisely relate to oppression targeting me and people around me? Oppression shames, pathologizes, convicts, degrades, dismisses. I have learned that I need to be grounded in myself and community, surrounded by love, as I relate to the oppression of the world around me and within me; otherwise, it can swallow me. This is part of both yogic and Buddhist teaching: the importance of sangha. We need community to mirror back our strongest selves. We need community to commiserate with. This is how humanity has survived, and how any group of people survives oppression: by strengthening from within.

The resilience we find in self-care practices necessarily impacts the resilience of the community as a whole, and as energetic beings we can sense the strength and vitality of those around us without words even being shared. Daily practices of yoga, meditation, eating well, sleeping at least eight hours each night, and spending time with beloveds are not just things that are "good to do" or that make me "healthy," but are actually core strategies that ensure my survival. Seane calls these "nonnegotiables." They are the practices I need to do each day so that I can do what I am here to do most skillfully and powerfully. These practices allow me to remain strong and vibrant, open, and kind.

As we engage in self-care practices, we are also taking care of the collective body—our partnerships, our families, our communities, our organizations, our projects, and the world. It is important to balance self-care with collective care. Some of us are socialized to take care of others first, often at our own peril (particularly people socialized as girls and women, as well as folks of color). Others are constantly invited to put ourselves first and not do vital care work (often related to male privilege and white privilege). During the course of the 2020 pandemic, I watched women and people of color get off the sidewalk, make room for other folks, whereas white men rarely moved, expecting others to make space for them or imagining themselves to be invincible. We must be watchful of our own positionality in the work of self-care and collective care, and endeavor to correct historical imbalances.

Due to the law of interdependence, when others around us are healthy, including plant and animal beings, we are necessarily healthier ourselves. This is called vicarious resilience. We need each other to be healthy so that we can learn from and be inspired by that, and also so that we can fall apart and be held by others, allowing our own vulnerability to be present.

Queer communities need to recognize that we internalize the trauma present in our world, work environments, and communities, and we recycle it onto each other. Many leading organizations run by queer people of color, such as Black Youth Project 100, the Black Visions Collective, and the Audre Lorde Project, engage in collective care practices, having learned lessons of what happens when this isn't prioritized. Mindfulness practices are so important—to catch our attention, our thoughts, our view of things before they manifest into words and actions. We can cultivate the skills and find the resources to transform our trauma into love, courage, and integrity. We need to do this to end suffering in our own lives and the suffering in the world.

There's a story that has been retold by many Buddhist teachers over the years about a time when the Buddha was confronted with an angry person. To this man, it seemed that there were too many people traveling from the city to his village, and each had something to sell or teach. Impatient with the bulging crowd of monks and villagers, he shouted at the Buddha, "Go away! You just want to take advantage of us! You teachers come here to say a few pretty words and then ask for food and money!" But the Buddha was unruffled by these insults and remained calm. He politely asked the man to come forward. The Buddha asked, "Dear sir, if you purchased a gift for someone, but they did not accept the gift, who then owns the gift?"

The question took the young man by surprise. "I guess the gift would still be mine because I was the one who bought it." The Buddha replied, "Right. You have just cursed me and been angry with me. If I do not accept your curses, if I do not get insulted and angry in return, these curses will fall back upon you—the same as the gift returning to its owner." The young man then clasped his hands and bowed to the Buddha, acknowledging the lesson learned.

I love this story as an ancient teaching of how to interact with oppression—the Buddha teaches that we have the option to give it back, to refuse to internalize it, while still recognizing its existence. In part, I think that queer communities are very skilled at this, as we create chosen family, build our own institutions, create the world that we want to live in. This resilience is so powerful, and it's something that many communities that have survived hatred have learned to do.

The Buddha didn't tell the man that he was wrong or evil, he didn't even push him away; rather, he said, "This anger of yours, this hatred, you can keep it," in quite a loving way that not only set a boundary but provided a teaching to the deliverer of anger. How I can relate to oppression and those perpetuating oppression is an important inquiry! Can I allow someone who makes a condescending remark to me and my lover in public or calls security on me for being in the "wrong" locker room at the gym to keep their hatred? Under duress, we must increase our self-care practices and invite in community when we are threatened so that we can hold the weight together.

The greatest transformations from hatred that I have seen have been through personal relationships. It's often difficult, charged, potent territory—but I believe in this micro work for big change. Loving one another across difference leads those in power to leverage their privilege and those who are targeted to heal, forgive, and rebuild trust.

Through my mom's relationship with me she can love other trans people and care about the issues that impact us. Through relationship between white folks and people of color we can each heal from the deep wound of racism. Through my relationship with my beloved Lezlie Frye, I learn how to become an ally to disabled people, and she learns to trust a nondisabled person. This work takes willingness, practice, tears, integrity, courage, determination, and patience from all involved. It's hard work that many folks never do—a 2014 study found that 75 percent of white folks' networks are exclusively white, and a 2017 study found that 84 percent of people in the US don't know a single trans person.[2] Those in targeted communities may become exhausted in these relationships if the other party isn't willing to do the deep, continuous, and humbling work of self-study and self-education about communities that one is not a part of, challenging systems of oppression, taking accountability for microaggressions, and leveraging their privilege for the benefit of those with less power.

When someone in a privileged group *can* and *does* do these things, and the person in the relationship with less power has done enough healing to trust the other person, trust themselves to create boundaries and speak up about harm, and trust the other party to respect those boundaries, something amazing can happen. We see this in the victory won by the Domestic Workers Alliance and Jews for Racial and Economic Justice (JFREJ) in passing the first statewide Domestic Workers' Bill of Rights in 2010.[3] JFREJ members who employed domestic workers lobbied the state congress in support of the bill, alongside domestic workers. They did this due to many house parties and intimate relationship-building work between the two organizations.

Ultimately it is my spiritual work to change how I relate to the hate, violence, and injustice in the world. I must create boundaries that protect me from internalizing harm, while practicing compassion that allows me to remain sensitive to suffering around the world and in my own life. Holding on to anger and rage literally makes us unhealthy and creates harm in our lives—self-harm, harm of loved ones in our words and actions, and, inevitably, harm that manifests in our political work. We need to create space to attend to the grief, move the energy of the anger out, and then show up with wisdom and commitment.

Anger tells us, *pay attention!* Anger gives us the energy to do something, for something precious is being killed, injured, threatened, tarnished, taken, abused, polluted, appropriated, or harmed. Take note of the anger's energy and release it before speaking or acting, otherwise its fire may know no bounds and may hurt those close and nearby. For me, after the heat in my body has passed, after my jaw has loosened, after deep breaths are again easy to access, after the righteous story that I created and rehearsed in my mind has dissipated, then I speak. Then I do the change work. I make the call, I show up at the rally, I write the article, I raise my hand in a training.

We can shift how we relate to violence and injustice while still doing everything we can to counteract it and build a better world. We need that world to exist with us in it, still alive, the changemakers and visionaries healthy and vital—so *how* we do the work really matters. We want to do our social justice work in a way that is reparative, restorative, revitalizing, so that we're not worn out with broken hearts and broken bodies when the world we want arrives.

PRACTICE: TONGLEN MEDITATION

The Tibetan Buddhist *tonglen* practice utilizes the breath, thereby making the meditation a somatic experience. With the breath, we rehearse different phrases, shifting these phrases four times during the meditation; stay with each set for several minutes.

Find a comfortable seated posture and concentrate on the breath to center your attention. Your eyes may be closed or downcast. Bring your attention to your breath and for several minutes simply notice the inhale and notice the exhale.

In this practice, sit for several minutes saying inwardly with each breath, *breathing in love and breathing out love.* On the inhale, breathe in the love that surrounds you, and on the exhale, return that love to the world.

After some time, shift the words you repeat inwardly to *breathing in suffering and breathing out love.* Here we intentionally turn toward suffering, let it touch our heart, and return love rather than passing on the suffering. Empower yourself to be in relationship with suffering, while being purposeful to breathe out love.

If you become overwhelmed at any time during this meditation, look around and find three things unique to the space that you are in, take a few deep breaths, and reach your hand to the sturdiness of the ground beneath you. If you feel steady enough to continue, please proceed. Or you may choose to just pay attention to the breath again without any words and come back to the meditation another time when you are more resourced.

If you choose to continue, begin to shift the words again to *breathing in love and breathing out suffering*. Breathe love into your body once again, and let go of your own suffering—any armor you are holding, resentment, fear, or anger. Allow yourself to let it go and, perhaps, to forgive.

Finally, return to the original words, *breathing in love and breathing out love*. The breathing in of love here is the practice of gratitude—beholding and drawing in the beauty and brilliance of this world. The breathing out of love is the practice of generosity—sharing what you love and offering your love, time, resources, and attention.

When it's time to let go of the words, sit for a few moments with an awareness of your heart. Notice what is present. Take some deep breaths, open your eyes, and attend to the needs of your body.

COMPASSION: THE VIOLENCE STOPS WITH ME

In recognizing the preciousness of all of life, may we resolve to not add one single further drop of suffering to a world that already hurts so much.

—LARRY YANG

WHEN WE ARE faced with pain, we have the option to contract and close, resist, deny, avoid, and dismiss—or open our hearts and turn toward and tend to the pain. How we relate to pain in our lives can either worsen a situation or give it witness and meaning. If we don't do the work to heal from violence and oppression, examine the small ways that we participate in violence, and work to face and dissipate our tension and stress, then we run the risk of creating more harm and suffering. This involves in-depth spiritual work—examining somatic reactions in our bodies, investigating patterns in our minds, and considering any ways that our scars have created armor around our hearts.

Karuna, a Pali and Sanskrit word, means a quivering of the heart in response to pain, commonly translated as compassion. Compassion is the second Brahma Vihara, turning unconditional love and unwavering attention toward pain, struggle, oppression, and violence. Compassion is that soft quality of heart from whence tears come. Compassion knows only suffering and the end of suffering—it does not consider right or wrong. Compassion does not mean getting rid of pain; that is not possible—pain is inevitable in this human life. Compassion is cultivating a presence and tenderness toward pain. When we relate to it with friendliness and care, it is more manageable and passes more quickly.

I started teaching Trans Yoga in 2006 at the NYC LGBT Center, and it evolved into Yoga for All Genders, a class that ran at the Center until I left the city in 2014. When I opened Third Root in Brooklyn, we put many classes for specific communities on the schedule, and I gave Queer and Trans Yoga prime-time spots on Sunday afternoons and Thursday evenings in order to center this community. I began this class because I saw yoga as a tool for my community, and also because I had faced countless micro-aggressions in typical yoga studios and I wanted my community to have a different experience. I have now taught Queer and Trans Yoga workshops across the country and as a weekly class in four towns and cities, and I am gratified to see many queer and trans yoga teachers holding such classes in their own communities. This intersection of queerness and yoga practice would not have been possible without me turning toward my wounds of exclusion, harm, and harassment within yoga studios and trainings. One of my yoga students, Caro Marr, once said on a retreat, "There is a portal to the divine in anything, and thus, there is a portal to the divine in everything." Any harm can provide insight into what is most precious and important, and therefore can lead to new visions and new creations.

If we are receiving hatred and fear from the world around us, how can we transform that into love? For many years, I thought that this meant loving other queer and trans people, which is a journey in itself, and an important one. Given that we have faced immense trauma and oppression, if targeted communities don't do the hard work of transformation then we perpetuate our fear, sadness, and anxiety onto those closest to us— our chosen families. We see this in queer community in factions created over issues like same-sex marriage, or divisions along lines of race, class, dis/ability, gender, and more, or community splits due to friends choosing sides after a breakup. The work of loving each other as a community is the work of sangha that Buddhism and yoga—and every spiritual tradition—point us toward. Work in community is profound, difficult, and important for individual and collective spiritual growth. Kazu Haga, a Kingian Nonviolence trainer, challenges us all in his book *Healing Resistance,* "If you are not struggling to love people, if you are not trying to build understanding with those you disagree with, then you are not really doing the work of building Beloved Community. The work of building Beloved Community is understanding that we're not trying to win *over* people, but we're trying to *win people over*. Historically, winning a war has meant defeating the opponent. There is a clear winner and a clear loser. The victory is *over* your opponent. But in nonviolence, there is no real victory until everyone is on the same side."[1]

After becoming a supporter of the Equal Justice Initiative in Montgomery, Alabama, I received their racial injustice calendar. On each day, or nearly each day, the calendar logs something horrible—a lynching, an arson, a murder, a rape. I knew about some of the events, but sadly, I can't say I knew about most of them, which is why I continued this practice for several years. I brought the calendar to my altar, and before each sitting, I read what had happened that day in racialized terrorism—what white people just like me had done to Black neighbors, business owners, community members, entire families, neighborhoods, and congregations. Some days, I would cry rivers of tears. Some days I would be shut down and stony, unable to take in the gravity. Some days, my resolve of anti-racism would deepen.

I read the calendar each day at the beginning of my meditation practice to enliven my practice, to remind myself that I'm not just sitting for me, not just reducing my stress or even just pursuing my own awakening. I am sitting to transform the harm enacted by my ancestors into accountability, reparations, and solidarity. I am not sitting to "save" anyone; I am not doing anyone any favors—I am sitting to reclaim my wholeness and my dignity, and that of future generations. I reviewed these horrific acts as inspiration to work diligently to water the seeds of love and not the seeds of hatred. We have seen what watering the seeds of hatred can look like.

It has manifested as white supremacy. We know where that road takes us. Reading the Equal Justice Initiative's calendar each day recommitted me to the ethical practices of Buddhism and yoga, and kept me watchful for slight and profound residues of fear, resentment, and hatred within me.

A challenging piece of the work of compassion is that of loving the people who have hurt me the most, working to forgive them and understand that the harm came out of their own confusion, ignorance, or pain. This applies not only to the very individuals who have hurt me but also to their identity in the world. For me, one such group is middle-class white women: I have been hurt by rejection of my trans identity by my mom, by her best friend who is a second mom to me, by feminist mentors, by lovers. I teach yoga, where 75 percent of yoga practitioners are women and 80 percent are white:[2] the universe is inviting me to grow, to take the harm I've received and, rather than add another drop, transform it into an offering. The universe is inviting me to grow to love not just the people like me but also the people who resemble those who have hurt people like me (as well as the actual people who have hurt me). The Buddha says that "hatred does not cease by hatred, but by love alone. This is an eternal law."[3] This demands that people facing oppression turn toward their oppressors, returning love rather than retaliating and perpetuating violence. Out of a love for this world, a recognition of the preciousness of all things, we heal our own wounds and work to love broadly.

"Your Greatest Wound Is Your Greatest Gift"

This teaching, offered by Off the Mat, Into the World teachers Suzanne Sterling, Seane Corn, and Hala Khouri, has allowed me to turn toward my pain with compassion and inquiry. Life is full of ten thousand joys and ten thousand sorrows, and our task as practitioners is to be present to it all, without attachment or aversion. "Your greatest wound is your greatest gift" encouraged me to work with my pain, sit with it, and gather insight from it, rather than deny, avoid, resist, or fight it—and I hadn't encountered this elsewhere in my life. Before I encountered this teaching, I thought of myself as "damaged goods" or "too messy." This teaching expanded my awareness, implying that everyone is wounded and that that is not a bad thing after all. I am not disposable because of the ways I've been harmed or enacted harm, and therefore neither is anyone else.

I include this teaching in this book because I see a lot of harm inflicted upon our own queer fellows within our own communities, organizations, and relationships. We create queer community out of protection and a beautiful intention of chosen family—a deep alliance to one another that can be stronger than blood for many. We face great violence in the world, from daily microaggressions to the real threat of murder for simply being ourselves. That is a lot to handle, and unless we stop to examine ourselves and our own patterns, assumptions, addictions, and wounds, then community is not going to be safe. I see queer people being judgmental of one another, excommunicating someone if they make a mistake, and being reluctant to forgive. In this reaction we loosen the bonds of community and create a hostile environment for some people. In turning toward our greatest wounds, this also involves holding space for one another to be messy, to work through wounds, and to move toward love, with patience and compassion—and regarding this as sacred work. We draw boundaries when needed, to ensure our own safety, but hold space for our own and each other's process.

There is a story of a mustard seed as a portal to enlightenment in Buddhism, where a woman named Kisa loses her only son. She is struck with grief and carries the dead child from practitioner to practitioner, hoping to revive him. Finally she meets with the Buddha, who tells Kisa that he can help her if she retrieves a handful of mustard seeds from a home that has been untouched by death. Many households are happy to give Kisa mustard seeds, but when she asks if anyone has died there, they all reply that in fact their house has seen death. Through this assignment given by the Buddha, Kisa realizes that her grief is common across the land, and she returns to the Buddha, becoming a student and seeking refuge in the dharma.

All of us have hurt someone. And all of us have been hurt by someone. This is something that connects us to all of humanity. My suffering may be different than my mother's, but it is suffering just the same. Since all human beings suffer, turning toward my own suffering turns me toward all of humanity. When I do the work to see my own wounds, fully, along with the shame and guilt that accompany them, it gives me the courage to see others' pain fully.

In Becky Thompson's book *Survivors on the Yoga Mat,* she notes how many survivors of trauma and abuse open healing centers and do social justice work; because of our own trauma, we want healing not only for ourselves but for all. Due to surviving the trauma, our compassion and understanding for all of humanity can be so much broader.

I co-founded Third Root two years after being fired for being trans from a natural food store owned by a yoga ashram in New York City. I had been out as trans for a few years at that point, and dressed in a tie and button-down shirt each day for work, gratified that I got to work with herbs and supplements and hone my herbal skills and knowledge within a yogic institution. I had many conversations with coworkers about pronouns and transphobia, inviting them out of harm and into alliance. At a three-month performance review, I was told that such conversations were "inappropriate" and "distracting." I was also asked intimate questions about my body, which I felt obligated to answer given the power differential, feeling that my job was on the line. At a partner's suggestion, after that meeting I met with a legal intern at the Sylvia Rivera Law Project, an organization in New York that exclusively serves trans and gender nonconforming people. Six months after that performance review, I arrived to work to find the store fully staffed. The assistant manager walked me outside, telling me they had filled the position with someone else and were letting me go. I was heartbroken that a business based on yoga, where staff answer the phones with "how may I serve you?" could inflict such harm. I felt humiliated, betrayed, and afraid of having few financial resources or sources of support at the time to rely on. I was filled with rage for being fired for being trans despite living in a city with nondiscrimination protections around gender identity.

I returned to the Sylvia Rivera Law Project, and a lawyer told me that although this law is in place, it is very difficult to prove discrimination and would involve time, money, and pain, and suggested that I let it go and not fight it. I did not know it at the time, but this was a pivotal moment in my life—from wanting to rely on laws and policy that supposedly protect oppressed groups of people to creating a worker-owned cooperative, where no one could fire me, and I could not fire anyone else, without a collective decision. Out of my pain and sense of helplessness at having no control at the yoga apothecary, I transformed the energy to create an institution where many people have a say in the day-to-day happenings and larger direction of the business, and where most of the worker-owners have complex identities of privilege and oppression.

Sorrow, stress, and trauma give meaning and purpose to our lives. Kelly McGonigal, a scientist at Stanford University, notes that those who have experienced two to four traumatic life events have more resilience and happiness than those with either fewer or greater traumatic life events.[4] This is not to say that we would wish trauma on anyone because it will give them meaning and happiness! Emmanuel Jal, a hip-hop artist and a former Lost Boy from Sudan, who survived a civil war and walked hundreds of miles with other children through the desert, sings "what doesn't kill me can only make me stronger, stronger. What doesn't kill me can only make me wiser, wiser," in his song "Stronger."[5] The trauma that I have survived gives my life meaning and importance, teaches me how to better live by wisdom, discernment, and compassion.

Part of healing my wound of being fired for being trans was starting my own business with others whose identities also made them vulnerable in a myriad of ways. At Third Root, we were all committed to a just working environment, and there wasn't a singular person who could terminate someone else's employment; instead, an entire collective made those decisions collectively. Additionally, the collective was accountable to the community in a way that the natural food store that I was fired from was not. In healing my wound, I co-founded an institution with worker protections and community accountability.

Freedom on the Inside

In 2015 and 2016, I taught two semesters of a fourteen-session course on Buddhism at Five Points Correctional Facility in Romulus, New York, a twenty-minute drive from where I lived in Geneva, New York. When my partner and I moved to Geneva in 2014, I signed up for several pen pal services with incarcerated people; aware that we were within a half-hour drive from five prisons, it seemed an opportunity for relationship. I had had many friends in New York who were involved in Critical Resistance, a prison abolition organization; I had trained with the Lineage Project to teach yoga in prison; and I was familiar with several prison education programs. I soon became aware of a college program at Five Points that was run by one of my yoga students, an English professor at the college where my partner taught. My student soon invited me to teach as well.

In the course that I taught, each three-hour session together we meditated at the beginning and end of class, I gave a dharma talk, and we had an activity and discussion related to the teaching. The students were engaged, eager, hardworking, and thoughtful. At the start of the class students arranged themselves starkly along racial lines, but both semesters, by our last session men of different backgrounds gave each other fist bumps, pats on the back, and nodding acknowledgments, having witnessed one another's pain and common humanity.

In a compassion activity, I asked everyone to write on a sheet of paper a great suffering in their life, with no details that would convey their identity, and to fold it up. I then collected the papers in a basket and redistributed them, asking the students to make sure that they didn't receive their own. Before opening the paper I asked them to pause and consider that they had something sacred in their hands: another man's suffering. Then I invited everyone to open the paper and read what was written silently, take it into their hearts, let it touch them, take deep breaths, and offer compassion to whoever this writer was. After several minutes, I invited each man to read aloud what was written. We heard, "I lost my mom and couldn't go to her funeral"; "I'm not there for my kid's first day of school"; "My kid's mom is trying to turn my kids against me"; "I am incarcerated for a crime I didn't commit"; "My mom gave me this disease"; "I killed my best friend"; "It's hard to raise my kids from the inside, and instill the values I want them to have."

We took a breath together after each one, and the room was gripped, beholding the suffering that we collectively held. After the ritual of reading aloud the suffering in the room, I invited the men to share whatever was alive and present for them. One shared, "I didn't write about being a father, but I am one. To all of you fathers in the room, each of you that wrote about it and those of you who didn't, I feel you." A bunch of men agreed, looking around the room with compassion for one another. Another man shared, "It was interesting that I got the one about addiction. I didn't cause this man's addiction, but I sold heroin in my community, leading to someone's addiction." His eyes filled with tears, and he finished, "To each of you in recovery, I'm so sorry." I told the students that in any room that we are ever in, there are these stories and this pain, largely unknown. When we can soften into that reality, it can enhance our relationships with one another, shifting judgment to understanding, blame to compassion.

I next invited the class to consider their resilience—what they've learned through their suffering that they might not have known otherwise, or skills that they've had to develop because of what they've been through. One man on the window side of the room stumbled with this one, saying, "I just don't get what good can come of a life sentence. I don't think anything can." A younger man raised his hand, asking me, "If I may?" I usually didn't allow students to give each other advice or comment on one another's stories, but I felt sincerity from this young man, and had seen his need to prove himself melt away during the semester. I nodded at him, and he turned to look at the man who had just spoken. "Man, look at you. You're getting a college education. You're making something of yourself *regardless* of your life sentence. You've been here twenty years and you're still at it! All us young guys come in here scared, and then we see someone like you. You create a model for us, man." My eyes filled with tears, watching one man show up for another. The first man, teary-eyed as well, looked the young man in the eye. "Thank you." Another man shared that he wouldn't kill someone again, but given that he had, he absolutely knew the value of each human life. "I didn't really know before, and that's how I could do it. Now I do, and I couldn't do it again."

The summer of 2016, after I taught these two courses, my partner received a new position in Massachusetts; I could no longer teach at Five Points. Before I left the area that summer, through the prison chaplain I organized a day-long meditation retreat. About ten men from my two classes joined the retreat. We committed to abide by the five precepts as we had in class and practiced Noble Silence, except during my dharma talk, meditation instructions, and their reflections at the end. The five precepts of Buddhism are the ethical practices observed within and outside of practice spaces, which include harmlessness, nonstealing, using sexual energies toward connection and healing, truthfulness, and moderation in intoxicants. Noble Silence is a practice found on many meditation retreats, in which retreatants commit to not communicate in words or gestures in the interest of the introspection of everyone. Similar to a residential retreat, at the Five Points retreat we alternated sitting and moving meditation. One man in a wheelchair wheeled back and forth, pivoting his chair with attention and grace, and others walked the width of the room, turned, and walked back for thirty-minute periods.

The most memorable part of the day was lunch. The chaplain had asked me if I wanted one of the bag lunches that the guys were having. I was familiar with the injustice of terrible prison food. I also reflected that it would illuminate division if I didn't eat the same bag lunch that everyone else was having. I said yes, and asked if I could bring in some snacks, as I had some dietary restrictions—implying that they were for myself. The snacks were for the retreatants, for later in the day. I brought a couple of my favorite chocolate bars, and tomatoes and strawberries from nearby farms.

I gave everyone a half hour for lunch, we continued to practice Noble Silence, and I instructed them in mindful eating. In each bag was a bologna and American cheese sandwich with a squeeze of mustard on white bread, a tiny four-ounce container of apple juice, and a Red Delicious apple. At the end of the day, one of the men shared, "Mindfulness of eating made me realize how terrible our food is here. Maybe in this case, mindfulness is not wise?" We discussed that question for a while. Another retreatant shared, "This was much more time than we get for lunch, and I didn't have to protect my food. I could be present to it. When new guys arrive here, we tell them, 'eat now, chew later'—the faster you eat, the less chance it will get stolen. This was the first time I feel like I really *ate* lunch in two decades." I think about that share so often at retreats: how in our retreat inside a violent institution, in our cement-walled chapel with a wooden Jesus from the '70s hanging over us, paint flaking off his beard, the men could really eat. They trusted that the others would abide by the precepts and not steal or harm, and rather than using up mental energy toward stealing one another's food, they could be present to eating.

At the end of the day I took out my "snacks." I passed them around—two strawberries, three cherry tomatoes, and four squares of chocolate each. I asked everyone to eat this food mindfully, in Noble Silence, as well, and I watched these men be overcome by flavor and smell and a child-like delight. I saw them take tiny bites from the strawberries, making them last. I had thought that the chocolate was my best offering, but afterward one retreatant shared, "You said that was a what? Those little round things?" A tomato. "Right. No, I've never had something like that before. That was exquisite." Another said, "Strawberries! I haven't had strawberries since my twelfth birthday. You really took me back, professor." People locked up don't get to eat real food, real food that in upstate New York grows right next to the prison—the rural area is a mishmash of prisons, vineyards, liberal arts colleges, corporate dairy operations, and farms!

We begin to heal ourselves by investigating our wounds, our past, and getting curious about how those wounds impact our reactions to the present moment, how that open or healed wound influences how we see the world as safe or frightening. Working to heal my trauma with cisgender straight men and let men into my heart heals generations of trauma. This is not just my own trauma, but that of anyone who has been harmed, assaulted, or killed by a masculinity that manifests as power over others, control of others, unstated abuse of others. As Nikki Myers says, "the only way is through." We have to embrace our past as individuals and culturally, wherever we come from—including the pain—in order to access our power, our gifts. The ground of heartbreak is important, because something has touched our heart and the vast sky of wisdom within us that exists beneath our fear. If we go toward the wound, we go toward the wisdom.

PRACTICE: COMPASSION MEDITATION

In this compassion practice, allow yourself to feel any sorrow present in your heart and in our world, following Ruby Sales's invitation, "Where does it hurt?" You will offer the below phrases to someone you love who is suffering, to yourself and your own suffering, to an unfamiliar neutral person who is suffering (whom you have heard about in the news or seen in your neighborhood), and to someone who has created harm to you or in our world (a difficult person). Over time we aspire to attune to the pain of the world, pushing nothing away; we build our capacity gradually through patience and determination.

First, choose a comfortable seat. The recommendation is to be seated upright, in order to be energized in your practice, but knowing that discomfort is bound to arise. This is the first act of compassion: taking your seat with integrity and vulnerability.

Now begin offering the following phrases, first to yourself, and then to a benefactor, to a neutral person, to a loved one, and to a difficult person, working with each person for several minutes. Try to remain present to whatever arises, perhaps rage, grief, or empathy.

This is a moment of suffering.

Suffering is a part of life.

May I turn toward this pain / your pain with compassion,

And allow this unwanted experience to expand my heart and deepen my practice.

After some time, let the words come to a close and sit quietly listening to your heart. When it feels like the right time, you might bring your hands together in front of the heart and bow, honoring your practice, honoring all those who also diligently work to open their hearts alongside, before, and after you, and honoring the teachings and the ancestors of these teachings.

FORGIVENESS:
RELEASING THE BURDEN

Forgiveness is giving up all hope of a better past.

—LILY TOMLIN, by way of Gina Sharpe

AT A FORGIVENESS-SPECIFIC meditation retreat in 2013 at the Insight Meditation Society, Larry Yang opened by saying, "Everyone here has been hurt. And everyone here has hurt someone." That opening provided a great relief to me, as if for my whole life I had been trying to prove that I was not someone who hurt others. I could own the ways in which I'd been hurt and had been denying this factor of my own humanity—that I am bound to hurt someone, perhaps not intentionally, but definitely at least unintentionally. I longed to no longer be hurt and to no longer cause pain to others, and I had learned through social justice work that this was the goal, *this* was justice—the absence of pain. The Buddha would have had a nice chuckle at that one. Pain is part of the human condition—that's the first thing he taught!

That statement by Larry Yang created a sense of cohesion in the room— we shared this experience of harm. Naomi Shihab Nye writes in her poem "Kindness," "Before you know kindness as the deepest thing inside, / you must know sorrow as the other deepest thing. / You must wake up with sorrow. / You must speak to it till your voice / catches the thread of all the sorrows / and you see the size of the cloth."[1] Jack Kornfield says, "Everyone who loves is hurt in some way. Everyone who enters the marketplace gets betrayed. The loss is not just your pain, it is the pain of being alive."[2] At the Insight Meditation Society, Larry Yang opened me right up and primed me for the important and memorable work of that week.

The practice of forgiveness involves forgiving ourselves for the ways in which we have harmed ourselves in thought, word, or deed; considering the ways in which we have each harmed others and asking for forgiveness; forgiving those who have harmed us; and forgiving the First Noble Truth in Buddhism—that *dukkha* (a Pali word meaning suffering, difficulty, stress) exists in the first place. Buddhist teacher Gina Sharpe teaches that forgiveness is "giving up all hope of a better past," in the words of Lily Tomlin— that changing history is impossible, so how can we accept our particular history as a way of moving on? Gina Sharpe invites us into equanimity with this quote, to be with the way things are and the way things have been, because although the play-by-play can be rehearsed and analyzed, we can't have a do-over. Given that the past can't be relived, our best option—that is, the path that leads toward individual and collective freedom—is to intentionally and directly let it go, to forgive.

Forgiving does not mean condoning harm: harm is never "right" or "just." If I do not forgive the harm caused to me, the pain will continue to live on inside of me. Of course we would not have chosen acute moments of harm and ingrained, institutional forms of harm. Forgiveness is never about saying that what happened was okay, or that it needed to happen in order for some spiritual growth to occur. Inevitably in forgiveness practice, anger arises. Should you encounter such anger in your own practice, I hope that you will reference the second chapter of this section on anger and sustainability.

Nonviolence is an ethical practice of both Buddhism and yoga because it is integral to creating a healthy society. We each are responsible for that. Forgiveness is about how we respond to and heal from the violence that has happened, given that it never should have happened in the first place. Within forgiveness practice, there is room to say "ouch, that hurt," "that was painful," and "that was unskillful." In the practice of forgiving, we make room for those who have caused harm to claim their mistake, to move out of shame and guilt (which is their own pain) and into accountability and transformation. We hold the fullness of their humanity, that someone is more than their worst actions. When someone creates harm, a part of their humanity is shut off, which is painful for everyone involved.

Gina Sharpe also teaches, "We don't need to keep carrying that shit around." The forgiveness practice that I practice works in four directions, beginning with acknowledging and turning toward pain. I allow myself to feel the ways in which my body has stored pain, to breathe into all of the surrounding emotions, and to see the stories that my mind has made up about the pain—likely stories of righteousness, resentment, guilt, shame, or rage. Feeling the pain and allowing room for grief and rage are essential in an authentic forgiveness process. Then, if it feels right, I begin to offer myself forgiveness for harm I've caused myself and others, I offer forgiveness to the individuals who have caused me pain, and I ask for forgiveness from those whom I have caused pain, knowingly or unknowingly. Lastly, I offer forgiveness for the First Noble Truth, a component added by Larry Yang: that pain and sorrow are an inevitable a part of this human life. This forgiveness is directed toward large, systemic pain such as police brutality, the separation of immigrant children from their parents under ICE custody, and climate change and its escalating impact on the most vulnerable communities. Forgiveness in each of these directions is profound work that can shift the trajectory of our households, neighborhoods, cities, and world, witnessing pain, processing it, releasing its energy, and learning necessary practices so as to not repeat and perpetuate pain.

Mpho Tutu van Furth, daughter of Desmond Tutu and a pastor and author with a PhD in forgiveness, says that forgiveness involves a shift in identity. "You get to tell your own story in your own words and to say that the perpetrator is not the person who describes who you are," Tutu van Furth says. "Because when somebody injures you, it's as though they define you. If somebody slaps your face, they then define you as the person whose face can be slapped. When you are able to forgive someone for slapping your face, what you're saying is 'No, actually, I'm better than what you say I am. I am not the person whose face can be slapped. I am the person who can say, "that doesn't happen. I'm done with you, or I'm done with being in this kind of a relationship."""[3] Forgiveness involves setting boundaries and trusting that both parties are so much more than one moment of harm.

It is my work to forgive the abusers of my grandmother, my mother, my ancestors, my friends, my lovers, my community, those different than me, and those whose lives follow similar tracks. I must forgive those who preach homophobia on the New York City subway, those who murder trans women of color, those in my own life who have doubted, denied, or dismissed my own truth of who I am. I could remain enraged at all of these people, historic and contemporary, who cause harm. Remaining enraged would not enhance my freedom or well-being, but rather create greater suffering for me, as well as toward those who encounter my bitterness and resentment.

Forgiveness involves vulnerability and nobility, courage and presence, and it moves on its own timeline; you can't force it. I set my intention on forgiveness, for if I cannot offer forgiveness in this moment, I hope to be able to in the future. I incline my heart toward forgiveness. Forgiveness is different than condoning wrongs, and different than reconciliation. Forgiveness is the personal practice of release; it may never lead to reconciling with those who have hurt you or those you have hurt.

As with compassion practice, initially we offer forgiveness toward those who are annoying or irritating, those who have created harm but on a small scale: my neighbors who put trash in their compost bin, which is then left on the street and not picked up because it's not compost. Eventually we aspire to grow our forgiveness muscles toward those who have perpetuated the greatest harm—not to let them off the hook but to grow our own hearts to be that vast. I am inspired that Nelson Mandela worked to forgive and befriend his guards at Robben Island, Pollsmoor Prison, and Victor Verster Prison. It is hard to enact cruel punishment on your friends! He was so effective that his former guards attended his presidential inauguration and funeral. There are stories of mothers of young men who have been murdered who have forgiven, befriended, and even adopted their sons' killers, committed to the idea that love heals whereas shame and blame beget more harm.

A support of forgiveness practice is to consider the suffering that might come from the inability to forgive. What does the future of a held resentment look like? I had an example in my Grandma Helen and Great-Aunt Dorothy. Growing up, Dorothy was the "chosen daughter" of their father. In his eyes, Dorothy could do no wrong, and he offered her gifts no one else received. My grandma was left out, denied, and deprived. Within this context, my grandma courageously asked for a dress from her father for a dance when she was a teenager, and he told her no and shamed her for even asking. This created a rift in the relationship between Dorothy and Helen for the duration of their lives, and patterns carried out in each of their individual lives. My grandma rarely asked for what she needed or wanted, and she became distraught and angry when people didn't deliver her unspoken wishes.

When I was seven or eight years old, my mom, my grandma, and I went to visit my aunt and uncle and new cousin Renee in Seattle for a week. I was trying to connect with my new cousin and also offer time for the adults to spend time together, so I spent hours taking care of Renee. As we were packing up to leave, my grandma said to me, "I didn't even get to hold my new grandchild very much because you were holding her the whole time." I was so surprised, as I had been trying to do some babysitting and she hadn't communicated her desire to hold Renee more during the entire duration of the visit. I told my mom about the interaction, and she expressed familiarity with my grandma's resentment and an exhaustion at encountering it when it was too late.

My mom inherited the pattern and handed it down to me, and I have spent years diligently unworking it. Luckily for me, I have a partner who, based on her own lived experience as a disabled person, is very clear on what she needs and communicates that easily and directly, for otherwise her needs would not be met and that could have grave consequences. Lezlie's clarity and communication surprises me, even angers me sometimes, but it's a wonderful teaching and a counterbalance to my family's pattern, one that I want to disrupt for my own benefit and that of my child and all those I interact with.

Although my grandma and Great-Aunt Dorothy were close, this tension erupted often—my grandma resentful and Dorothy guilty—and neither had the skills and will to have a heart-to-heart about their father's actions and the harm caused. At one large family Christmas Eve party, which my grandma and Great-Aunt Dorothy always attended as the grandmothers of the family, they had another fight about it. They were in their late seventies and early eighties. Their inability to account for harm or ask for and offer forgiveness for decades created suffering for each of them for sixty years!

What if they had forgiven one another, and their father, decades before I came along? What would have been possible? I wonder if Dorothy could have allied with my grandma when she had asked for a dress and their father had refused. Perhaps Dorothy could have refused gifts that her siblings didn't also receive. Perhaps she could have asked for what her siblings wanted and offered it up once the gift was received. I wonder if my grandma could have approached Dorothy, asking for help, rather than bottling up her embarrassment, defeat, and rage for decades. I wonder if my grandma could have spoken to her father about her feelings, or if that was unsafe and she was protecting herself. I wonder if my great-grandfather was cruel. What if, unable to change the situation, Dorothy and my grandma had talked it out, and my grandma had forgiven Dorothy in their teenage years? Or what if my grandma had taken that wound into an intimate relationship or friendship and healed it, speaking her needs and desires? My heart breaks at thinking of my grandma bearing that weight for decades; I can feel her hurt.

Forgiving One's Self

There is a pervasive cultural notion that the way to improve yourself is through force and harshness. We are hard on ourselves; we have all kinds of unkind narratives running through our heads. We all make mistakes! In forgiving one's self, we forgive ourselves for the harm we have caused ourselves and others, knowing that we did so out of pain or ignorance. One of my students at Five Points wrote, in a reflection on forgiveness, "Look, this isn't easy ... the exploration of one's inner self takes time and proper guidance as well as the ability to bounce back from failure, because you gonna fail!"

This is humbling, right, but perhaps also freeing?

In our humanity, we make mistakes. We create harm. We hurt our-selves. Rather than relating to that with shame, blame, and guilt, can we turn toward it with compassion and attention? If we relate with shame, blame, and guilt, further arrows will be fired, creating further avoidable pain. In teaching forgiveness over the last ten years, many students have told me that self-forgiveness is most difficult. We hold ourselves to high standards that don't make room for our humanity. In a book I read my child called *I Am Human,* it says, "Being human means I am not perfect. I make mistakes. I hurt others with my words, my actions, and even my silence."[4] I wish I had read and been taught that when I was two!

I forgive myself for becoming controlling with food I ate and the exercise I did when I could not control or impact the bullying happening around me in high school. I forgive myself for not telling someone about the bul-lying. I forgive myself for not coming out to my grandma before she died, afraid of her rejection, willing to abide in allowing only a part of myself to be known. I forgive myself for the mistakes and errors I've made in social justice organizing, and at Third Root in particular. I forgive myself for the mistakes I've made in friendships and partnerships. In forgiving myself, I allow myself room to learn and grow. Some of this work takes more deter-mination and patience than others, but I have never regretted forgiveness. It always opens doors to possibilities that I could not have imagined.

When I was a junior in high school, a few friends and I were bowling and met four boys from a nearby town. We paired off and began dating. My best friend dated a boy named Dusty. My boyfriend was Mike, a young man with woodworking skills, kind and unimposing. I didn't know him well, he held a lot in, but he was fun and kind. I knew that his father was incredibly harsh with him, and that he would have preferred to live with his mother hours away. After several weeks I realized that I was not into him as a boyfriend and we were better suited to be friends. We went skiing and I decided to tell him on the ski lift. It seemed cruel to string him along pretending, and I wanted to be honest. He skied off after I told him. I called after him, "Wait, we can still be friends and ski together!" He shouted back to me, "Don't worry about it!" That evening I got a call from Dusty. He asked me if I was sitting down. I sat down. He told me that earlier that afternoon,

Mike had hung himself in his garage. I told him what had happened earlier in the day, and he said, "It's not your fault." My mom held me in a long hug once I got off the phone. Later that week, Dusty told me not to contact Mike's family, that they were angry with me for breaking Mike's heart. I knew several stories about Mike's dad from Mike, that he was a formidable force, and kept my distance.

On Monday at school, my counselor called me into her office because she had received a call from Mike's school about his death, and that he and I had been dating. The counselor was a friend who knew me well and helped me survive high school. I thought I was fine and just wanted to pretend that nothing had happened. She made me stay in her office all day. The truth is that I was numb and shut down. One hour I had been on the ski lift with Mike, and the next hour he had hung himself. I didn't have a narrative about it; I didn't have much of anything to say.

A week later my three friends who had dated Mike's friends attended the funeral with me a few towns over. When we arrived at the funeral, the students from Mike's high school stared at us, not sure who was the one who had broken up with Mike. I felt the blame in their eyes; the tension was palpable. I listened to story after story of Mike, learned a lot more about him, and grieved more deeply the loss of his life. Soon after, the couples of my friends and Mike's friends dissolved for various reasons. I know that part of it was our collective inability to acknowledge the pain of Mike's suicide and be thoughtful and caring with one another through it all.

The forgiveness I have offered myself for this formative romantic experience has been layered. I first had to learn how to feel its impact—in my body, in my heart, in the way that I engaged sexually and romantically. I don't feel a need to forgive myself for breaking up with him; that honesty is important. I have forgiven myself for not knowing the impact of the breakup, or the greater difficult context of his life. For years I did not break up with dates and lovers, even if the relationship was noticeably deteriorating. I have forgiven myself for not knowing Mike better, for not understanding all the pressures in his life. I have forgiven myself for not understanding how much people can invest into romantic and sexual relationships.

I have worked with forgiving Mike's dad for his harshness with his son, and the greater school community for not being a greater refuge for Mike. I have forgiven my own school community for not holding me tenderly, outside of the counselor's office. And I have worked to forgive a world that can be so painful that sometimes people cannot continue to exist within it.

When we forgive, we open doors of wisdom. I learned that I have no control over anyone but myself. I learned that difficult circumstances at home make one precarious and delicate; they need to be approached with great attention and care. I learned that a community can crumble if we don't turn toward the pain directly, courageously, and heal it. I learned why the ethical practice of *Ahimsa* (harmlessness and lovingkindness) comes before *Satya* (truthfulness), because the truth can hurt; rather than not telling the truth, or being cavalier with it, deliver truth with kindness and care for the receiver.

Letting Go of the Need to Be Right: Asking for Forgiveness

To ask for forgiveness demands courage, humility, and swallowing pride. It can mean letting go of "the need to be right," as Swami Jaya Devi says. It means admitting that you made a mistake. We work to be with it and recognize it, rather than covering it up, ignoring it, or denying the pain caused. Really, you've got nothing to lose. Asking for forgiveness is a practice of connection, of realignment on the path of love. It gives space for those whom we have hurt to have their feelings and perhaps to drop the burden of those emotions—if not now, then in the future.

Apologizing has a different energy than asking for forgiveness. In giving an apology, there is an admission of wrongdoing, a sense of taking responsibility, but it has an energy of disposal, of putting the apology upon someone whom we've hurt and demanding that they accept it. Forgiveness is an ask, a question, an open request, internal work done in our own hearts. We reckon with our own actions and face ourselves—"damn, I did that." We may or may not actually go to the person we've harmed—that is the external work of reconciliation. Someone accepting an offer of forgiveness is their own business, their own spiritual work of forgiving harm done. In asking for forgiveness, we are showing that we care about the person and our actions. We enable the hurt one to heal through the admission of our carelessness and ignorance, and to be empowered and self-determined in their own forgiveness process. Asking for forgiveness is like the opening of a gate. We learn from our mistakes through examining them.

At an LGBTQ meditation retreat a few years ago, my ex, my current partner, and I were all in attendance. My ex and I had been in a three-year open relationship, moving toward having a child and a farm on her family's land, when I met Lezlie. We had both made mistakes and caused harm in the midst of negotiating my relationship with Lezlie, and our relationship had ended. I believe I acted with integrity at that time, and I know that nevertheless I caused pain. When I heard that my ex would be present at the retreat, I was angry and frightened. Angry that a mutual friend hadn't told me until an hour or two beforehand, and frightened about difficult dynamics between Lezlie, myself, and my ex amid the silence of the meditation retreat space. I wanted a lovely retreat experience, and this felt like work!

Once the retreat commenced, I tried to open to the experience. I paid close attention to sensations and the movement of emotions through me, and I tried to practice kindness through both giving my ex space and holding doors open for her. It was a retreat practicing Noble Silence (no spoken words, no body language, no reading or writing, no eye contact), so interactions were subtle, which was healing in itself—we could be together but not need to negotiate our interactions in the same way. And I could practice kindness and compassion in almost a stealth way—no one had to know!

At the retreat, it was intense to be in close quarters with one another, which had happened before but being together in an LGBTQ-specific retreat felt different, held by the river of dharma. It felt appropriate, at an LGBTQ retreat, to have the opportunity to (silently) work through the pain of the breakup and the areas where I had not been skillful, and also recognize the pain of my ex, grapple with how Lezlie got ensnared and harmed, and hold my injuries tenderly as well.

One of the precarities of queer community is having to be in relationship with ex-partners, because the community tends to be small and tight-knit.

We are often forced to share spaces with people we have harmed or who have harmed us, as lovers, colleagues, or friends. This is part of the reality of being queer—there are few of us, and we often rely on community-specific spaces for socializing, professional opportunities, romance, and more; thus, there is often history and drama in these spaces. I know that in any queer space I enter into there is an invisible web of history with one another—people avoiding each other, hard feelings and hurt, solid relationships that have survived fires, new colleague relationships that are thus far untested, flirtatious energy pointing toward relationships in the future, and silence, resentment, and shutdown. This demands a lot of our communities, to hold all parties in compassion, to accept multiple truths at once—and we aren't always skillful. At the retreat, just being in close proximity with my ex, and in silent practice within community, a softness emerged.

As my heart opened and my attention became more astute throughout the retreat, I decided to write a letter to my ex on the last evening there. I recognized the ways that I had been unwise or unskillful in our relationship and breakup, without making any excuses or providing context or explanation. I tried to not make excuses for why I'd made the decisions that I had, but rather stay present to the impact of my actions, not whether they were in the "right" or not. Afterward, when reflecting upon the retreat with Lezlie, I told her about the letter, and she asked if I would share it with her. I did so, and she began to cry, because, she said, some of the same patterns were present in our relationship and the ways in which I was not skillful with her.

A component of asking for forgiveness is releasing any expectation that it will be held in a specific way. I sent the letter to my ex, and a year later she emailed me. Her email was short and direct. It was not reconciliation. My practice was in the asking, in the willingness to put my mistakes on the page, and it would have been harmful to myself and to her to expect anything specific to come of that. There is a surrender in the process of forgiveness—perhaps nothing will change other than our own hearts! My ex appreciated the responsibility that I'd taken for my actions and wished me luck in the future. If I had expected my ex to respond right away and say "I forgive you," or if I'd had a storyline in mind, I would have been bound to be disappointed. The reception is not the point—it's about the work that I did within myself, to work toward healing and reconciliation but let go of it happening in that moment.

Offering Forgiveness: A Vision of Healing

The next direction of forgiveness is to offer forgiveness to those who have harmed us. In so doing, we aspire to accept someone in their full humanity: their mistakes, their vulnerability, their ignorance, and their potential to change and grow. We recognize that someone who creates harm is not at their best in that moment but is acting from their own hurt. Like some of the other practices, offering forgiveness does not have to mean proximity to someone who has caused harm, or imagining that they behave differently. Welcoming someone into your heart is not the same as welcoming them into your home. You can forgive at a distance, where you feel safe and protected from the person who inflicted harm.

A person's decision to forgive is up to that person—they have to arrive at that place on their own, they have to be ready to let go and open their hearts toward someone who created harm. Someone else could suggest it or offer up the teaching, but an authentic offering of forgiveness comes from a person's own heart. If one is not ready, forgiveness can seem ludicrous or even dangerous. Feeling the emotions of grief, disappointment, betrayal, sadness, and anger are all prerequisites for offering forgiveness. If these emotions are not fully felt before one turns toward forgiveness, it can erode the process and compromise its authenticity.

Once the feelings about a situation or relationship have been substantially felt, cried, sweated, or screamed out, then assess whether you are ready to forgive. Perhaps you need some space from the situation, or perhaps you need greater support before making your heart more vulnerable. Madeline Klyne says that forgiveness "ennobles the heart." It makes the heart stronger, broader, more vast, and deeper than before. The aspiration is to forgive all the hurt—again, not to make it "okay," but to free your heart from that pain and be able to love deeply and vastly.

One of my bullies once sent me a friend request on Facebook when the platform was in its infancy. In seventh grade, this schoolmate had sat behind me and tickled my neck, made fun of me to other girls, and called me gay. At my bully's lead, girls moved away from me in the locker room (thinking I was gay and checking them out and punishing me with isolation), refused to room with me on school trips, trashed my locker, wrote "faggot" on my locker, and resisted my attempts at friendship. I had two kind and courageous friends for those six years. This particular classmate's bullying continued and gained traction through high school. Some of my worst bullies were recognized as the leaders of the school—basketball team captains, the loudest and most influential voices in the hallways. I wrote my schoolmate back on Facebook messenger, saying, "I know this is just a silly social media platform and not real life, but even in this format, I don't want to be friends or let you into my life. You bullied me relentlessly for six years and encouraged others to do the same. I have forgiven you; this is not punishment. I genuinely hope you have a lovely life with joy and love. Given your behavior when we were young, I'm declining your friend request." I didn't know what would come of that, but a week later she responded, saying that she hadn't been aware of her impact on me and that it made sense that I didn't want to be friends. She apologized, and also wished me a good life.

The end result of forgiveness is never prescribed and can't be anticipated. There may not even be an "end result" but rather a meandering pathway with opportunities and possibilities along the way. When I recognize and attend to old wounds and offer forgiveness, doors that I never even saw continue opening.

Forgiveness toward the First Noble Truth

Turning toward forgiving the First Noble Truth is heavy lifting. We are invited to turn toward the most profound difficulties facing humanity—things like climate change, the prevalence of domestic violence and childhood sexual abuse, police violence, government corruption, environmental disasters—and accept that this is the way things are, and the way things have been. Being with the truth of how things are is healing in itself; there is a reason honesty and transparency are practices spanning spiritual traditions! When we can do that, freeing ourselves from denial, avoidance, resistance, and dismissal, it frees up our capacity for vision and imagination.

Pain and sorrow are an inevitable part of this human life, the Buddha taught. They touch all of us, although they impact some folks more harshly and with generational affects. Swami Jaya Devi's teacher, Ma Jaya Sati Bhagavati, a Jewish woman from Queens, said that "pain is pain." It's not helpful to compare pain—in that process we inevitably disregard one person's pain, perhaps our own, thinking that it's not as great as someone else's. There is always someone in more pain. Going down that line of thinking prevents us from seeing and being with the pain in front of us—it locates our attention elsewhere; it's a distraction. At another time, we can turn toward that pain.

And pain is not distributed equally; it impacts marginalized people at greater rates. Black birth parents are three times more likely to die in childbirth than white parents.[5] Fat people have higher unemployment rates, are less likely to be hired and less likely to earn a high salary, and earn fewer benefits than slimmer people.[6] Forty-five percent of undocumented people do not have health insurance, which can lead to undiagnosed or untreated conditions or extremely high medical bills when they do seek treatment.[7] Black young men aged fourteen to twenty-four were the targets of 25 percent of police stops in New York from 2014 to 2017 despite comprising only 2 percent of the population.[8] Only 19 percent of disabled people were employed in 2019 compared to 66 percent of nondisabled people.[9] More or less, across arenas of pain and sorrow, marginalized communities fare worse.

The directions of forgiveness can be overlapping. As a white person, I must forgive myself, forgive my ancestors, ask for forgiveness from impacted and traumatized communities, and forgive the larger history. Remember, forgiveness is an internal practice, different than reconciliation or making amends. The US has a violent history of racism that continues in explicit and implicit ways. My colleague Rhonda Magee tells us, "The fundamental cost of [racism] is material, creating and reinforcing walls that block access to necessary resources—including education, money, health care, and political power—rendering the vulnerable all the more so."[10] To really be present to the immense harm that has been created and is actively perpetuated daily and to live into a different future invites us toward forgiveness practice. Perhaps a different future demands forgiveness. Rhonda Magee reminds us, "We all learn the rules of race, the often subtle messages about who matters more and who matters less."[11] The link between the recognition of how racism works and where it shows up and creating a just, safe, equitable world for all of us may be forgiveness. Buddhist teacher Ruth King tells us, "Racism is a human capital system driven by greed and fear—a fear of losing power and a fear of payback."[12] Forgiveness is not the only pertinent practice here, for healing racism also involves examining greed and fear—and cultivating their antidotes, generosity and courage. But I don't think we can move toward healing and justice without forgiveness.

Anti-racist activist Jardana Peacock suggests, "White supremacy's biggest win is to disconnect people from knowing where we came from. For white folks, there is simultaneously a message that we belong everywhere and yet a disconnection from learning or valuing the roots of where we actually come from."[13] I must forgive my own white family and ancestors, who were a complex constellation of enslavers, Quakers, settlers of Indigenous land, members of the Ku Klux Klan, and members of the International Workers of the World. There are many ancestors' stories that I do not know, and I grieve that loss of knowing my people. Perhaps there were abolitionists and allies whose stories have disappeared. My lineage contains a terrible history, but it is my history, and I have no other. If I hate these ancestors, I continue to allow my heart to hate, and that does the world no good and creates no progress toward racial justice.

I am angry that my blood relatives enacted harm and cultivated hate in their hearts, and I am full of immense sadness when I consider the victims and survivors. Forgiveness does not condone their actions. In fact, I find that forgiveness demands that I know my ancestors better, seeing their many harms alongside their humanity. I write and speak about this history and the corrective actions I can take with family members to engage in racial justice work and deepen my practices to break the chains of violence. Forgiveness is an aspiration toward harmlessness, and it frees up psychic energy that can be used to promote goodness, care, and ethical practice in the world.

In forgiving my ancestors, I also forgive myself for my own mistakes and reproduction of white supremacy, and I commit to generations of reconciliation. It took five hundred years to get into this mess in the United States, and it will take at least that long to heal. My hope is that I can contribute to healing, rather than further harm, and that my child and his children continue in the legacy of healing and justice, onward toward another five hundred years. This takes great awareness from moment to moment to be incredibly intentional with my words and actions, and I am grateful to this practice for its support and tools.

A student in my Five Points class wrote, "When we all open our hearts up, and endeavor to be honest and nonjudgmental of others, we start to change our mindsets. When we truly empathize with other people's suffering, we start to feel compassion for them. This can lead to bringing communities closer together, in which everyone's welfare is protected. When nobody feels left out or alone, the world is moving in the right direction. When communities care about the mental health of [their] people, and show compassion for them, we reduce the number of suicides around the world."

In forgiving myself, I turn toward the history of pain to know exactly what I am forgiving myself for. I am not condoning it; I am recognizing it and grieving how things are and how things have been. In forgiving myself, I release shame and guilt, which doesn't serve anyone, and allow myself to grieve, to contribute to the ocean of tears caused by this history. In forgiving myself I recognize that my participation in racism and settler colonialism interferes with my deep desire to create a world of equity and justice. In forgiving myself, asking for forgiveness, and learning behaviors and actions that create racial justice, I craft space for relationships and collaborations to create that future together.

Gay Buddhist teacher Eric Kolvig teaches about changing the mind from abiding in suffering to abiding in happiness. Aggression is fed by aggression but is disarmed by warmth and generosity, and turning toward the pain is an important aspect of moving past it.

In "A Christmas Sermon on Peace" in 1967, Martin Luther King Jr. said:

Somehow we must be able to stand up before our most bitter opponents and say: "We shall match your capacity to inflict suffering by our capacity to endure suffering. We will meet your physical force with soul force. Do to us what you will and we will still love you. We cannot in all good conscience obey your unjust laws and abide by the unjust system, because non-cooperation with evil is as much a moral obligation as is cooperation with good, and so throw us in jail and we will still love you. Bomb our homes and threaten our children, and, as difficult as it is, we will still love you. Send your hooded perpetrators of violence into our communities at the midnight hour and drag us out on some wayside road and leave us half-dead as you beat us, and we will still love you. Send your propaganda agents around the country, and make it appear that we are not fit, culturally and otherwise, for integration, and we'll still love you. But be assured that we'll wear you down by our capacity to suffer, and one day we will win our freedom. We will not only win freedom for ourselves; we will so appeal to your heart and conscience that we will win you in the process, and our victory will be a double victory."[4]

In this final direction of forgiveness, we invite ourselves to be with large, complex, intricate difficulties—to turn toward them, growing our capacity for presence and awareness. This practice invites us to educate ourselves on large issues we may be less aware of, a prerequisite for holding them in our hearts. And, given this awareness, we commit ourselves to a different world to live into. We cannot create a different, better world if we cannot be with the pain of how things are and have been.

Sylvia Boorstein is often quoted as saying, "This is what is happening. I wonder what will happen next." We turn toward what has happened and what is happening—the ten thousand joys and the ten thousand sorrows—and practice kindness, compassion, and forgiveness and wait to see what happens. All over the world, formal processes of forgiveness and reconciliation are being enacted—between the Hutus and Tutsis of Rwanda, between Israeli and Palestinian children, between the descendants of enslavers and the descendants of enslaved people in the United States. This work is deep, powerful, and promotes healing. It is moving out of harm's way, refusing to escalate, and valuing all of humanity as precious, followed by a practice of curiosity.

When you practice forgiveness, you tap into the wisdom of humanity—a practice of healing that transcends culture, identity, or religion.

Forgiveness is difficult, important, exciting work. What is possible when we learn what we need to learn from a circumstance where harm was created and admit to the pain fully? What comes after that? What comes of those who were harmed, if they forgive? What comes of our relationship to one another when pain was caused, is recognized by all, and is forgiven? What future does that allow us all to live into?

PRACTICE: FORGIVENESS MEDITATION

As offered by Eric Kolvig during early LGBTQ retreats of the 1990s in the Insight tradition. The fourth direction was added by Larry Yang.

Make sure you are in a comfortable seat, able to be present and open. Begin to feel into your heart center and what it is holding today with curiosity. Consider how resourced and balanced you are today and if you can turn toward great suffering or only the small stuff. When you are ready, begin offering forgiveness in the following directions, allowing time at the end to sit with what arose.

Offering forgiveness toward yourself:

For any way that I have caused harm to myself,
Through judgment, action, self-blame, indifference,
Knowingly or unknowingly,
In thought, word, or deed,
I forgive myself.

May I allow myself to be a student of life and to make mistakes.
May I forgive myself,
And if I cannot do so in this moment,
May I be able to forgive myself in the future.

Asking for forgiveness from those you've harmed:

For any way that I have caused harm to you,
Knowingly or unknowingly,

In thought, word, or deed,
I ask for your forgiveness.

May you accept me with my imperfections and mistakes.
May you allow me to learn from my actions.
I ask for your forgiveness,
And if you cannot forgive me in this moment,
May you be able to forgive me in the future.

Offering forgiveness to those who have harmed you:
For any way that you have caused harm to me,
Knowingly or unknowingly,
In thought, word, or deed,
I forgive you.

May I allow you, too, to be a student of life and to make mistakes.
May I recognize your humanity, in the midst of my pain.
May my forgiveness soften any difficulties between us.
May I forgive you,
And if I cannot do so in this moment,
May I be able to forgive you in the future.

Directing forgiveness toward a greater suffering (destruction, tragedy, violence, abuse, war):
For any way that I have been unable to be present with,
And respond skillfully to,
The pain and suffering of our world,
My own pain, and that of others,
May I hold the pain with compassion,
And offer forgiveness for the way things are, and the way things have been.

A TUSSLE
WITH EQUANIMITY

The scripture doesn't say anything about the next moment.
—LARRY YANG

EQUANIMITY, *UPEKKHA* IN Pali, is a warm acceptance of reality as it is, rather than how we might like it to be. Rather than aversion, attachment, or indifference, there is a quality of acceptance and acknowledgement of the way things are and the way things have been. When I offer equanimity to others, this involves a gentle acceptance that someone else's freedom is up to them, beyond my own control. The Buddha described the equanimous mind as abundant, exalted, immeasurable, without hostility or ill will.

Equanimity invites a willingness to be with this moment as it is, without any notions of what it "should" be, with a sense of wonder, awe, and curiosity. Equanimity is the last practice of the Brahma Viharas, considered to have a balancing quality to compassion, sympathetic joy, and lovingkindness, with an understanding that everyone's liberation is only and solely up to them, that no matter how much I wish compassion and love upon you, your freedom is yours. This is an unclouding of the mind, giving up our stories and ruminations, that may be unnecessary. We are encouraged to trust and surrender. A student of mine at Five Points wrote in a reflection on *upekkha*, "The Buddha taught about equanimity in order to bring a sense of balance to those who could adhere to his teachings. He wanted people to understand that in the blink of an eye, we could experience the many extremes of pain and pleasure. The Bible teaches that the sun shines down on the wicked and the just all the same—life happens to everyone."

My spiritual practice is constantly informing, intersecting with, and challenging my social justice work, and vice versa, and I have had a consistent tussle with this teaching of equanimity: to accept things as they are, rather than how I might like them to be. I have been engaged in social justice work for several decades, and I have been taught to constantly challenge the existing reality—a reality full of racism, homophobia, fatphobia, misogyny, ableism, ageism, and other forms of oppression.

A related teaching from Jaya Devi is, "It's not about you." When someone is behaving or speaking unskillfully, it comes from their pain and confusion. It's not actually a reaction to you—it's not personal. This doesn't mean that challenges, critical feedback, or suggestions are not worthwhile—they are, when they come from a place of connection. If it's not about me, if it's not personal, then I can access spaciousness and equanimity about the moment, which allows me my creativity and compassion—to hold the pain or solve the problem.

It is our task to love, to love hard, to weed out everything that stands between us and a regular embodiment of love; yet, at the end, our task is to let it all go. There is such a wisdom in letting go—for many of us, there can be an idea that we didn't do enough or aren't enough in who we are; equanimity transcends that judgment. We show up in our lives as we want the world to be, and then we let go, and see what happens. Sylvia Boorstein asks, "I wonder what will happen next?" out of a curiosity and sense of awe—nothing is scripted; everything could change.

Zen master Seng-tsan taught that true freedom is being "without anxiety about imperfection."[1] Shunryu Suzuki Roshi said, looking out on a crowd of thousands of students: "Each of you is perfect the way you are ... and you could use a little improvement."[2] The idea is that the yearning for perfection actually takes us away from full presence with the imperfection of this moment. In our relationships, organizations, and social movements, can we accept imperfection? Can we accept mistakes as a basic condition of life and at the same time continue to engage with crafting a better world?

At exactly the same moment that a crow landed on a palm tree, a coconut fell, a story from the Yoga Vasistha tells us. Now, was that coconut going to fall anyway, and it didn't actually matter if the crow landed there or not? Or did the coconut fall precisely because of the minute impact of the crow landing on the palm tree? This story is a koan—a spiritual riddle. We will never know whether it was the crow's doing, but we must show up in our lives as though we are making coconuts fall again and again.

In the practice of equanimity, we endeavor to embody a vast perspective and wisdom. I think of Julia Bennett, a coworker of mine at Third Root and a Black queer woman in her sixties. Her politic is fierce; she is on the side of justice always. She is constantly learning how to ally with various communities, and she is very involved as a healing force in her own Black community. In moments when difficult things would happen in the world—from the verdict in the trial of Eric Garner's killer to the death of Leslie Feinberg, Julia would always be touched by it and let her emotions flow, tears streaming down her cheeks. Julia often said, "I'm just tryin' to be grown." She embodied equanimity and being a student of life—an acceptance both of reality and of all the work that there is for us to do in the pursuit of liberation for all. When I become overwhelmed, caught up in "change now!," I try to channel Julia's energy, her fortitude, trust, equanimity, and commitment.

Social Justice and Equanimity

How do I accept reality as it is and not as I would like it to be, given all of the oppression and injustice in the world? And what would it look like, I wonder, to engage more equanimity in our justice movements? One quality of a bodhisattva that the Buddha discussed in the *Karaniya Metta Sutta* is to be "easily contented." What would it mean to be "easily contented" (as the Buddha suggested) as a movement, an organization, a collective—or even as organizers, fundraisers, educators for justice?

I know that it is helpful to my nervous system, and to my spiritual path, to accept reality as it is. On the other hand, the existing reality breaks my heart. There are countless things that break my heart in our society today, which is what led me to become an activist when I was nineteen—to do what I can to change things. To accept reality—to accept *this* reality, to accept this reality *as it is*—feels like a condoning of the injustices in the world and an apathy toward social change.

There is an urgency to every social movement that I have ever been part of: racial justice, men working on misogyny, food justice, organic farming, environmental justice, queer liberation, and healing justice. This urgency drives us to not only change *the next moment* but also to change *this very moment*. This is not only unsustainable but unattainable. If racism exists in this moment, then it exists in this moment. Urgency creates an endless to-do list and a dynamic within social justice work that is stressed, rushed, and perpetually unsatisfied. This has led to social justice idealizing the martyr: someone self-sacrificing to the movement, working every possible moment of every day, showing up at every protest, negating their own needs (and often that of their families), not ever resting. I have seen the harm of this ideal break bodies down, because we don't take care of them or release the tension that is building every day from the work that they are doing. We need to rest; we need time away—and that actually nourishes our social change work.

Tara Brach says, "We are uncomfortable in our lives because everything in our lives keeps changing—our inner moods, our bodies, our work, the people we love, the world we live in. We can't hang on to anything—a beautiful sunset, a sweet taste, an intimate moment with a lover, our very existence as the body/mind we call self—because all things come and go. Lacking any permanent satisfaction, we continually need another injection of fuel, stimulation, reassurance from loved ones, medicine, exercise, and meditation. We are continually driven to become something more, to experience something else."³ The work of equanimity is counter to our instincts; it forges a new neural pathway. This perpetuation of craving, of always wanting more or wanting different, doesn't create happiness or liberation—it is a cycle of suffering. The patience, kindness, and spaciousness implied in the teaching to accept this moment is important for all of us—and important to social justice work in particular. It has allowed me to take a breath; otherwise I would resist and just keep moving.

After consulting many teachers on this question of equanimity and social justice, Larry Yang answered my inquiry about equanimity in a satisfying way. He said, "The scripture doesn't say anything about the next moment." We can accept things as they are in this moment, and we must, for it already exists—while at the same time trying to prevent harm in the world in the next moment. It helps me be with the oppression, the powerlessness, the despair present in this moment if I can feel empowered to change the next moment. I can offer compassion to this moment in human history if I know that I and comrades that I work with are doing everything we can on personal, interpersonal, and institutional levels to create justice and equity.

Sangha is a key component of equanimity work: none of us can do this work alone; we cannot face all of the suffering in the world in isolation—we need community, we need backup. Spiritual traditions involve community for support on the path, for assistance when we are discouraged, for guidance when we are lost. The sangha helps us be present in this work and feel that we are not alone, which allows us to personally continue and find inspiration and support in one another. Having spiritual community is also a way to practice how we show up in the rest of our lives. We know that whatever is inside of us will show up on our cushions and on our mats, and it will show up in whatever relationships we have. In a sangha, we share spiritual practices and commitments that create a container of trust for the individual work that we do—trust that we don't necessarily have in the rest of our lives.

"The scripture doesn't say anything about the next moment" encourages me to work on my own racism, misogyny, internalized gender norms, ableism, and countless other prejudices, to recognize culturally embedded patterns before they externalize into words, action, and livelihood. The current moment is the result of our collective thoughts, words, and actions, so how do we all make the shifts on the inside that then shift what we say and do in the world?

Dream It, Build It, and Let Go

For five years in yoga spaces, I would study with a teacher, try out another yoga studio and try to push its politics, and get denied or dismissed. A quote by R. Buckminster Fuller continues to guide me when confronting how something in the world is unjust or oppressive: "You don't change things by fighting the existing reality. You change things by creating a new model that makes the old model obsolete."[4] The moment that I stopped fighting the existing reality was a moment of moving into my power. I met Green Wayland-Llewellin, and we co-founded Third Root together in 2008, knowing that the kind of spaces where our own communities could heal and practice wouldn't exist unless we created them. We created a space where social justice and healing were intertwined and held as equally important and interdependent, a business that offered acupuncture, herbal medicine, massage, yoga, Buddhist studies, an herbal education program, and health education.

The creation and sustenance of Third Root was not an easy one—we began as a worker-owned cooperative owned by seven beings of diverse identities and backgrounds, with different life experiences and trauma, and different relationships to authority. We owned a business in a capitalist world where profit is prioritized, yet we tried to practice economic justice among ourselves as co-owners, with our employees, and with clients and students. It is no small thing to have our economic survival dependent on one another across lines of race, sexuality, size, gender, disability, and age; everything about our experience with any of those aspects of our being comes up, and the dial is turned up, because our survival as individuals and that of the business is at stake. At times I was overwhelmed or resistant, thinking, "No, sexual harm can't happen here! Fatphobia, transphobia, and racism between collective members is unacceptable!" At different moments, profound harm surfaced or was created. One summer I turned to Susan Raffo, an experienced organizer and healer in Minneapolis. She told me that this was the work that I'd signed up to do—to address each aspect of our history and to create a different way of being in the world. I'd signed up to practice healing justice, she told me, very deliberately. The only way is through.

As a co-owner of Third Root I had to show up, regardless of the conditions. I had to continue to show up alongside people of vastly different backgrounds. I had to show up on days when I was overcome by the grief of the world or how the injustice of the world manifested in our small collective. I had to show up when Hurricane Sandy hit, when a co-owner's dad had a stroke, when a coworker's nephew was shot, or when I was in a space of heartbreak in my personal life. I had to foster equanimity with all of the calamity and beauty that would arise at Third Root, a willingness to be with imperfection, while the greater community was watching us and turning to us. This demanded equanimity from all involved. At moments, collective members left, or shifted their relationship to Third Root, and I had to sit with my disappointment and grief, learn about why they made the decision to leave, and continually try to craft a responsive and brave space. When we discovered that our accountant had made errors on our taxes, or that due to our business structure our personal tax liability was great, I had to continue to show up, continually learn how to build a successful and sustainable community space.

The greatest letting go was in 2014 when my partner received a job at a small liberal arts college in upstate New York. We had to move, and I had to relinquish my ownership, trust my co-owners to carry Third Root on in their own way, and allow it to evolve without me. Although grief surfaced for me in this transition, it was surpassed by a great amount of joy. Third Root had become so much to so many people. We had inspired folks who were queer and/or people of color to become healing practitioners themselves, and some returned to practice at Third Root! It was a blessing. It had allowed me to build my work as a healer and then work outside of Third Root and meet colleagues in the greater yoga world. It was time to follow Lezlie's dream, to invest in that—for I had lived my dream.

The entire process included when Lezlie accepted the position—telling my business partners that I was moving on, telling my regular students that I was leaving Brooklyn, receiving payment for my portion of the business— was a practice of equanimity. I could hold on and create more suffering for myself and others, or I could let go and accept the moment. I fired up my equanimity practice—to be with feelings as they came up, to go with the moment and not fight it, to cultivate curiosity: What will it mean for me to do the work that I do in a small, rural, western New York town? What possibilities lie ahead for Third Root? How will the surrounding community shift? Equanimity practice created an easeful transition to a new period of my life and gave me faith in the wisdom of equanimity.

The Eight Worldly Winds

A young student of mine at Five Points wrote, "No one in this world experiences only gain and no loss, only pleasure and no pain. When we open to this truth, we discover that there is no need to hold on or to push away.

Rather than trying to control what can never be controlled, you should come to the balance of acceptance." The Eight Worldly Winds of pain and pleasure, gain and loss, fame and disrepute, praise and blame are a central teaching of *upekkha* within Buddhism. The Buddha tells us that these winds will touch our lives no matter what; it is part of the human condition.

This teaching gives me great relief, having been inundated with the message that a goal of life is to create a life of only praise with no blame, only gain and no loss, only pleasure and no pain. What a setup for suffering! When I experience the loss of another dear one in queer community to suicide, I remind myself that loss is inevitable. When I experience the gain of buying a house, I enjoy it, while reminding myself that there will be loss as well. When I receive praise for being a white ally to communities of color, I take that in, while reminding myself that I will also be blamed for not doing enough, for saying the wrong thing, saying too much, or saying nothing. When I experience the pain of loneliness from being a new parent in a community where I have shallow roots, I remember that both pain and pleasure are part of this life.

In 2014 I attended Nikki Myers's Yoga of 12-Step Recovery (Y12SR) training and was struck by how she introduced herself. Nikki often introduces herself in this way—telling the whole story, not just the glittery, shiny parts. She maintains the same tone throughout, conveying respect and acceptance for each part of her path, as tangled as it has been. She says,

> It has been a big journey to reintegrate all parts of myself—to accept without judgment all the various experiences that make up my whole—and come to radical self-acceptance. I'm a drug addict. I'm an alcoholic. I'm a codependent. I'm the survivor of both childhood and adult sexual trauma. I'm a love addict. I'm a recovering compulsive spender. I'm a yoga therapist. I'm a Somatic Experiencing practitioner. I'm the founder of Y12SR. I am the mother of two living children and one deceased child. I'm the grandmother of five. All of this is true, and I say that with gratitude and grace. I've discovered that if I exalt one part of myself and diminish another, I create a separation that becomes a war inside me, and that's the antithesis of yoga.[5]

I love Nikki's bold embrace of her whole self, conveying no regret, shame, or blame. This has been her path. As a teacher, I often find that when I share the tough moments of my life, and how I came back to love, balance, or trust, *that* is what is most useful for my students. Seane Corn has encouraged me to come into deep relationship with all parts of myself, to work through shame and guilt and come into a full embrace. Seane knows firsthand that when you lead, your flaws, ignorance, and mistakes are more visible. She taught me that when I am unafraid of everything being seen, I am actually safer than if I were to tuck things away and pray that my full humanity will not be witnessed.

The Buddha has said of disrepute that when it arises, we can ask, "Is this true?" If it's not true, it's not true, and we can let it go! If it is true, what a gift it is for something to be pointed out to me that I need to work on and heal or shift. The person who pointed it out, whether over social media or in person, publicly or privately, gracefully or angrily, is a teacher in that moment.

Amita Swadhin's work through their production *Secret Survivors* and their organization Mirror Memoirs, and their willingness to be so public about their history as a survivor, has invited me to also see that history as a source of connection and fuel for social justice work. I have worked to embrace being a survivor of incest as a child. I know that I am not alone. Almost half of all trans people are survivors of sexual violence, alongside a third of cisgender women and a sixth of cisgender men, and the numbers are even higher for most groups of people of color.[6] Amita writes in their biography on the Just Beginnings Collaborative website,

> *My dream is that we will come to see child sexual abuse in the same way we used to think about other forms of discrimination and violence that were once completely taboo to discuss—for instance, against HIV+ people, against LGBTQ communities, and against people seeking abortions. In my lifetime, we have moved from a culture of such profound shame and stigma that directly affected people could barely utter their truths, to now, when we have multi-million dollar infrastructure, organizations large and small, and highly visible grassroots movements that have achieved significant progress on these issues. We have faced other intractable social problems and achieved real progress. Ending child sexual abuse is possible. There is no problem we can't tackle through collective power, with directly affected people leading movement building efforts.[7]*

Through compassion practices we come into deep relationship with the pain of our world, and through equanimity we accept that this is the reality that we are working with; this is the way things are. James Baldwin wrote, "Not everything we face can be changed. But nothing can be changed that is not faced."[8] Of course we would not have chosen pain, but when it arises we can work to be present to it.

The winds are inevitable; they will blow and pass. When fame lifts me up or disrepute smashes me to the ground, I remember the tattoo written on my left forearm: "This will also change." I am reminded of a Taoist tale of a farmer touched by the winds. One day a farmer's two horses run away. His neighbor comes over, and with his hand on the farmer's shoulder, says, "Oh, this is terrible!" The farmer gently nods and says, "We'll see." The next day the horses run back with three other horses, and the neighbor comes over to celebrate. "We'll see," says the farmer. The next day the farmer's son is training the wild horses and gets bucked off, breaking a femur. The neighbor comes again, and says, "This is terrible!" The farmer, again, tending to his son, says, "We'll see." The next day members of the army come, gathering up able-bodied men to fight, and his son can't be recruited due to the injury. Each time something arises, the farmer holds it with an openness, curious about what will come next.

In my own family, when something arises, I have taken on the words of the farmer. Our housing inspection on our new house reveals mold in our basement. We'll see. The day care feeds our sniffly young child a sugary snack, when they know that we're a sugar-free family. My tomato plants' leaves roll up, but seem to still produce tomatoes okay. My testosterone runs out and Utah's coronavirus cases are on the rise. My mom can't visit because she doesn't have the time to do the necessary quarantine to protect our family with my partner's compromised immune system, but it's been a year since we saw her now. We'll see.

Those words remind me not to anticipate what the future is based on any present occurrence, but to just be with what is present right now. The Eight Worldly Winds touch our lives. It's unavoidable. Equanimity practice invites us to be even-keeled and aware of what is before us at any given time. When we are in reactivity—*This can't be happening! No, no, no, no!*—we rile our nervous systems up, turning on our sympathetic system, the fight-or-flight response. In that state, imagination and dreams don't matter. We're trying to survive. Sometimes that's all that we can do, and it is truly miraculous sometimes to just survive. But in survival mode, we don't dream. From a position of awareness and acceptance, wisdom and vision arise, so that we can powerfully construct a pathway toward a world without prisons, a world without childhood sexual abuse, a world that takes responsibility for the climate crisis and adjusts our ways of life so that we all can live together on this planet. When we are grounded in an understanding of how things came to be this way, and an acceptance that this, exactly here, is where we find ourselves, we can better get ourselves out of trouble. Our creativity, imaginations, vision, and dreams are then unleashed.

PRACTICE: EQUANIMITY MEDITATION

Find your way into a comfortable seat. Take five to seven deep breaths, breathing and sighing out through the mouth. Consider any of the Eight Worldly Winds that is blowing you around right now. Pain, pleasure, gain, loss, fame, disrepute, praise, or blame. Remind yourself that this is part of the human condition—these winds are inevitable. Invite yourself to feel into your experience with whatever has rocked your boat recently as you continue breathing deeply.

When you are ready, begin to offer these phrases to yourself, offering them again and again for a set period of time, perhaps five to ten minutes:

This is what is happening.

May I learn to be with reality as it is, rather than how I might like it to be.

May I be present to the comings and goings of life.

Next we turn our equanimity practice toward that which is going on for people around us. Equanimity isn't passivity but rather a warm acceptance of the way things are. In offering equanimity out in different directions, we remind ourselves that each person is in charge of their own liberation; despite our care, awakening is up to them.

Offer the following phrases to people in the categories of benefactor, neutral person, loved one, and difficult person, turning toward the Eight Worldly Winds that may be manifesting in their life and throwing them off-kilter. Work with each category of person for a set number of minutes, setting a timer for yourself if you like.

I care for you, but I cannot stop you from suffering.

May I hold your joys and sorrows with equanimity.

All beings are owners of their karma.

Their happiness or unhappiness is dependent on their actions,

Not upon my wishes for them.

WE ARE FABULOUS:
AN INVITATION INTO JOY

Me must love what is uniquely trans about us.
—LAVERNE COX

We are neurologically transformed by whatever we practice.
MADELINE KLYNE

"DRINK YOUR TEA slowly and reverently, as if it is the axis on which the world turns—slowly, evenly, without rushing toward the future, live the actual moment. Only this moment is life," teaches Thích Nhat Hanh.[1] The practice of mudita, or sympathetic joy, is about cultivating a sense of gladness or taking an active delight in life; it's about rapture, a sense of spirit, belovedness, timeless presence. Mudita is the third practice of the Brahma Viharas, directing our love toward beauty, pleasure, success, and delight. Mudita is about appreciating the good times without becoming attached to them—knowing that everything that arises will eventually decline but while the going is good, celebrating and enjoying it. We can take joy in the pleasures, comforts, and success of our own lives, and also that of others, and we are invited to enjoy simple things with intensity.

Mudita is a focus on the good, on what is working, without becoming attached, as everything we love will eventually change. The only wise relationship to pleasure is unattached appreciation. We want the goodness, the passion, the beauty, to last—but it won't. Our task is to enjoy the beautiful people around us as long as they're around, to cherish the wise words of elders for as long as they are with us, to pause and notice the beautiful fall leaves or snowfall or sunset, to listen to the beautiful voice of our favorite musicians. Mudita encourages us to find magic. To pause to witness it and take it in. The law of impermanence creates a sense of urgency for me—to do it now, enjoy it now, to not put something joyful off but to revel, cherish, be exalted now. Mary Oliver asks in her poem "The Summer Day," "Tell me, what is it you plan to do / with your one wild and precious life?"[2] Lucille Clifton invites us to celebrate her continued existence: "Come celebrate / with me that everyday / something has tried to kill me / and has failed."[3]

The practice of mudita is to think about every other living being as precious. The practices that strengthen mudita are gratitude, lovingkindness, and generosity. The obstacles to mudita are judgment, arrogance, comparison, insecurity, boredom, and envy. Strengthening our joy and diffusing the obstacles are both in our self-interest and create a healthier, stronger, even more creative community. This is a component of the intervention of Queer and Trans Yoga—to create spaces for our community to heal in body, heart, and soul. This is essential for our liberation.

Our judgment, arrogance, and insecurity do just the opposite—they alienate aspects of our community and make the internal environment of the community as a whole a frightening place—who knows when your politics may be judged, the way in which your breakup went down will fragment your friends and comrades, your fashion sense will be praised or critiqued? A friend on Facebook once wrote, "When I left radical queer community, my life got a whole lot better." This is cause for pause. It makes me wonder: How do we make our communities irresistible? How do we provide the skills and spaces for one another to heal?

The obstacles to mudita have to do with not being grounded in your own experience, and not being present in the moment. Judgment is thinking that people should do something differently, and involves a controlling element tinged with aversion. Comparison, relying on others' follies for one's own sense of worth, or always wanting more and different, takes us out of our own experience and out of the moment. Prejudice—really pre-judging—involves an immediate or unfounded dislike. Think of when you have brought that into a relationship—how did it go? Demeaning or wishing someone to be less is a waste of energy, and again takes us outside of our own experience. Envy is the hatred of others' happiness or prosperity—how does that feel inside yourself when you are in a state of envy? Are you suffering? Avarice is selfishness, greed, possession, and attachment, or the desire to keep goodness to one's self. Boredom is a lack of paying attention, a dullness, and a sense of separation. We can all see moments in our lives when we've put energy in these places, and I wonder, if you think back on such moments of boredom or comparison: How did that go? Did it lead to your well-being and happiness?

It's important to note that being in the present moment and grounded in your own experience is required for experiencing joy but quite frightening to survivors of trauma. In trauma, one's survival depended more on what others were doing than what was going on inside ourselves, and looking to the next moment for the dangers ahead. Being in the here and now for joy involves stability in one's life, not being under immediate threat. This does not mean that joy is not available to trauma survivors, but will involve some deliberate actions. In healing from trauma, for inspiration and a reminder of our own healing potential, we might place on our altars images of people who have survived immeasurable suffering, and have limitless love and a commitment to justice on the other side of that experience. Healing involves coming back to this moment, again and again, for longer and longer periods of time, gradually bringing awareness back into the body, and shifting awareness of others from one of hypervigilance toward one of trust.

Rumi says, "Let the beauty we love be what we do. / There are hundreds of ways to kneel and kiss the ground."[4] An aspect of my mudita practice is to read about the good news, the brilliant, creative, courageous things that people are doing in the world. Sometimes I need to read more about the good news than the bad, because it enlivens and enriches my own heart and mind. I subscribe to *YES! Magazine,* which publishes stories about victories, innovations, and successes—all the ways that justice and love are being manifested. I need to be reminded of how we live our love, and I think we all do. What each of us practices individually grows stronger within each of us, and what we practice in community grows stronger within the community.

Queer folks have a lot of joy; it's part of why I cherish queer community. We have traditions of drag, vogue, camp, theater, extravagant outfits, fun music. We are brilliant, cutting-edge thinkers, artists, and poets. We are in every facet of society, making space for ourselves and expanding the existing conventions. Purimshpil, an annual event put on by Jews for Racial and Economic Justice in New York, celebrates, amps up, and queers a Jewish cultural holiday, always incorporating the organization's social justice campaigns for the year—immigrant justice, workers' rights, abolition of the death penalty, and more. JFREJ states on their website, "Each year, the Purimshpil offers a powerful example of what can happen when we use our cultural abundance in our political organizing.... The shows have enlivened, enlightened, confused, and inspired JFREJ members and our friends and comrades."⁵ Events like this are essential components of our community health and resilience, to celebrate ourselves, to play, to enjoy.

In my workshops and trainings, I often give my students the assignment to write down something that they most appreciate about everyone in the room. Part of this practice is one of presence—have you been paying attention to the people and creatures and ecosystem around you? If so, it should be an easy activity to recall the goodness of each being. I then collect everyone's reflections and compile a list for each person about what is most revered and cherished about them by others in the training. Then I give each person back their list. In my Five Points class, students were moved to tears that they had been seen in their beauty. Many people in our world have not been witnessed in this way, and this activity can be reparative.

A practice of joy is to focus on similarities rather than differences, to use *us* and *we* rather than *they* and *them*. The default of our nervous systems is to value one's own group and devalue others, and this separation leads to violence and oppression. When we look for similarities we inevitably find common ground. Notice when your own mind goes to that place of *they* and *them,* and see what happens when you switch that up to be *we.*

When we consider having the eyes of a bodhisattva, to look upon all beings with love and compassion, as a community and individually, it might shift how we show up in community. At the annual LGBTQ meditation retreat at the Garrison Institute, we practice being in community with incredible age diversity—gay people in their eighties to queer folks in their twenties. The history and lived experiences held in that room is felt in the silence of the retreat. Given the practice of Noble Silence, we largely don't get to know each other's stories, histories, occupations, passions. Yet through being silent and mindful together, an intimacy is created. I become aware of when the man staying in the room next to mine awakens, and if he stays up late. I notice days when the person meditating next to me is settled, and when agitation is present. I notice who stockpiles cookies at lunch, who eats just one, and who takes none. I notice who drinks tea and who drinks coffee, and with how much cream.

The opportunity to be in community in this manner cultivates those eyes of the bodhisattva—after this retreat, my love and gratitude for queer people across generations is so great. Inevitably there are those in the room whose politics I would agree with and those whose politics I would not agree with. There are those present who have embraced me and those by whom I have felt excluded. There are close friends in the room and there are people who I wouldn't care to talk to. Over the three to four days together we each work to cultivate an open, loving heart, individually and as a community. That practice is sacred; it teaches me about how I want to be in community and how to create the communities that I want to be a part of.

Joy is essential to sustaining work for social change. If we only attend to the injustice, oppression, sorrow, and struggle, then we miss a lot of beauty and we are likely to burn out. When we spend time on joy, it gives us the fortitude to continue to build stronger, more just communities. Joy balances compassion. If we get too focused on sorrows, we die in their depths. Appreciation allows joy and sorrow to exist side by side. When our meetings are fun, when our rallies are a dance party, our movement grows.

Joy in Queer Community

Laverne Cox offers a profound teaching to trans community, and I think we cannot hear it enough, for it responds to histories of self-hatred and internalized transphobia from the world around us: we must love what is uniquely trans about us. Violence may be directed at us because of the things that mark us as trans, and it can be easy to hate those things, want to hide our identities, blame ourselves for the violence, or fester shame in who we are as trans people. This is a personal response to violence from the world around us, and it is reproduced within our communities in conscious and unconscious ways. If we don't uproot internalized oppression, we reproduce it and spit it all over each other. Healing Justice organizer and yoga teacher Yolo Akili writes, "If you are gay, and think that all gay people are manipulative, superficial, and can't be trusted, then that means you think that you are manipulative, superficial, and can't be trusted."[6]

This teaching that Laverne Cox offers is radical and transformative, creating individual well-being and collective well-being. The suggestion to love ourselves, our whole selves—that which is fabulous and sexy and that which is difficult and heartbreaking, that which is targeted and that which is celebrated. We must love each of ourselves individually for the light that we are, we must love one another individually as we are in relationship with one another, and we must love queer community broadly. I first encountered these words by Assata Shakur through actions led by FIERCE, a queer youth of color organization in New York City: "It is our duty to fight for our freedom. It is our duty to win. We must love each other and support each other. We have nothing to lose but our chains."[7] Living into this invitation, I must offer some love notes to queers.

I cherish queer community and have grown up in it since coming out at age twenty. I have been in many queer spaces that are incredibly loving, where I am thrilled when I look around at the fashion, innovation, passion, and politics that we collectively hold. We are beautiful, we are trend-setters, we are changemakers. It is part of who we are to challenge the norm, to live creative and resilient lives, to build community.

This may already be clear, but there is no one, unified, united queer community. There are many corners and sects of queer community, constantly shifting and of course impacted by dynamics of oppression—internalized, interpersonal, and systemic—in ways that magnify both trauma and resilience. Sometimes we are divided, and sometimes we are unified. Sometimes we break up with one another in friendships, relationships, organizations, collaborations, and sometimes we stick it out, re-create, adapt to changing lives and conditions of the world.

I am proud to be queer; I take strength and empowerment in that identity and wouldn't ever wish it any other way. I mean, I think I could make do if I weren't queer. I hope so. I honor the strength of our friendships—that we depend on each other in ways that often seem beyond the bounds of friendship and more like that of intimate partners, even when we aren't partners or lovers or don't have that history with one another. We take vacations together and care for homes and animals when friends are away. We are there for each other in sickness, graduations and awards, births, deaths, anniversaries, new jobs, injuries and assaults, organizations blossoming or shutting down.

When my partner graduated with a PhD from New York University, many more members of our queer family were there to witness her glory than blood family. When Black queer playwright and Freedom Train Productions founder Andre Lancaster died in 2018, queer family flew to the funeral from around the country to mourn the devastating loss together. When my child was born, queer families sent boxes of clothes, diapers, bottles, and blankets from Chicago, Minneapolis, and New York. I have donated to countless fundraisers for gender-affirming surgeries and supported numerous friends on the ground before and after. We are there for each other in a way that allows us individually and collectively to keep on keepin' on, and in this, again and again, we value and honor each other's rites of passage and lives as inherently worth living, which counters our dismissal or targeting in the world; we heal each other in the process of showing up. We love each other how we want to be loved, and in the process we continue to teach ourselves and validate in each other that we are worthy of loyal, strong, fabulous, passionate love.

I think of our radical politics and collective understanding of the world, grassroots power, and the shape and forms of those who hold power. I think of the books that line our bookshelves, from Audre Lorde, James Baldwin, Essex Hemphill, Michael Callen, Larry Kramer, bell hooks, E. Lynn Harris, Angela Davis, Leslie Feinberg, Amber Hollibaugh, June Jordan, Bayard Rustin, Octavia Butler, Dorothy Allison, Grace Lee Boggs, Roxanne Dunbar-Ortiz, and our anti-capitalist study groups that study these authors and thinkers together. I think of the fabulous, fun, radical queer organizations such as the Audre Lorde Project, Jews for Economic and Racial Justice, Southerners on New Ground, the former Queers for Economic Justice, the Trans Justice Funding Project, Sylvia Rivera Law Project, FIERCE, Idyll Dandy Arts (Ida), and Nolose, and the many other organizations with queer leadership such as Project South, Generative Somatics, Harriet's Apothecary, Northwest Justice Fund, Jewish Voices for Peace, Grassroots Global Justice, the NorthStar Foundation, Movement Strategy Center, the Icarus Project, Resource Generation, and the Center for Anti-Violence Education. Queers are leading profound changes within many religious communities, inviting the lineage into more profound practices of love and truth. We raise money for each other to make documentary films, go to yoga teacher trainings, have writing residencies, take activist sabbaticals. We do some great work in the world and make our communities a better place.

I have been held by my queer community, which makes me who I am today and contributes to my understanding of the world, of yoga and Buddhism, and of my place in it all. We can be a critical people, in the interest of creating something and living lives that are infallible, full of integrity, and just in thought, word, and deed. There are countless comrades and elders from whom I have learned skills in fundraising, organizational development, facilitation, writing skills, and so much more, and I draw on their decades of experience as queers in the world and live into the lineages of all those who created the possibility of their work, mentored them, and kept them alive. I am grateful to all the lesbian, gay, bisexual, queer, intersex, asexual, trans, nonbinary, gender nonconforming, and questioning people in the world and what we do and who we are that makes room not only for ourselves and those who come after us, but amid humanity more vastly, creating possibility and models for all people.

We Are Neurologically Transformed by What We Practice

If we hold on to our grief, rage, sadness, fury, disappointment, and betrayal, telling the stories again and again, we strengthen those neural pathways. If we let emotions move through us, which researchers have noted can happen in ninety seconds or less, respond to them with care, compassion, patience, and draw insight and direction from our experiences, we are healthier individually and collectively.

The scientific research on ancient practices of yoga and Buddhism is important and revelatory. Science has shown that we are neurologically transformed by whatever we practice. If we practice anger, our brains are hardwired to respond with anger. If we practice compassion, our minds are hardwired for compassion. The Buddha knew this. He said, "We are shaped by our thoughts, we become what we think."[8]

My friend and colleague Tessa Hicks Peterson teaches about post-traumatic growth—the concept that we can grow and become more vibrant and cognizant human beings as a result of trauma. Kelly McGonigal asserts that experiencing stress and trauma can bring meaning and energy to our lives; she found that believing that stress is bad for you is an independent risk factor. A University of Minnesota study of 30,000 people that assessed stress and mortality in people's lives found that 43 percent of people who had a lot of stress *and* believed it was bad for them had died eight years later. The study participants who had a lot of stress and did not believe it was harmful to them were the healthiest. Kelly McGonigal reported that stress hormones increase neuroplasticity so we can learn from difficult experiences, along with sleep, exercise, and meditation.[9]

What thrills me about this research is that it directly confronts the notion that many of us have had over time, that we are "broken" or "damaged"—that belief, by itself, is destructive. Edwidge Danticat writes, "She told me about a group of people in Guinea who carry the sky on their heads. They are the people of Creation. Strong, tall, and mighty people who can bear anything. Their Maker, she said, gives them the sky to carry because they are strong. These people do not know who they are, but if you see a lot of trouble in your life, it is because you were chosen to carry part of the sky on your head."[10] In the Japanese Kintsugi tradition of mending cracked or broken pottery with gold, the idea is that the "damage" is illuminated, a manifestation of the moment, of nonattachment, and of equanimity within changing conditions.

When we go through stress or difficulty, we can create resilience by considering who else is suffering and how we can support one another, considering sharing our experiences in service of helping others, asking ourselves "what do I want and need, and how can I create that for others?," and considering how members of a community under immense stress can also be a resource or asset to their community.

A pertinent term arising out of neurobiology is *vicarious resilience,* which is that one's individual resilience contributes to that of the collective. We build on each other's fabulousness, beauty, strength, courage, patience, and so forth. We can place our attention in a way that recognizes the human capacity to thrive, rather than just focusing on the tragedy itself. We can have gratitude for each other's life and existence as a queer person in the world (as well as our basic humanity), which is no small thing. Before even recognizing what we have done, said, or created, the fact that we exist, survive, and thrive as queer people is astounding and important to remember. Vicarious resilience is a way of creating the next moment—a method and reality of creating the next moment afresh, anew.

Kelly McGonigal teaches that community participation itself is a resilience practice. Queer people gather and find strength in one another; vicarious resilience is built into queer culture. We are stronger with one another, and the more we recognize each other's success, joys, and pleasures, the more these things arise and manifest in our own selves and lives. When we practice jealousy or resentment, that neural pathway grows stronger in our brains. When we tear each other down, when we act or speak from a place of anger, disappointment, shame, or blame, then that pattern grows stronger not only within ourselves, but within our communities. When we celebrate one another, cheering each other on, heralding each other's successes, we are able to take enjoyment not only in our own pleasure and success but also in that of everyone else in our community, and thus the joy within us multiplies.

Whatever we practice becomes stronger. If we practice judgment, our judgment becomes stronger. If we practice seeing the negative side, we become skilled at seeing the negative side in everything around us. If we practice generosity, kindness, and patience, that all becomes a stronger, more grooved neural pathway in our brains. Theravadan monk and Cambodian peacemaker Maha Ghosananda said: "The thought manifests as the word; / The word manifests as the deed; / The deed develops into habit; / And habit hardens into character. / So watch the thought and its ways with care, / And let it spring from love / Born out of concern for all beings."[11]

Gratitude

Gratitude involves an active counting of our blessings, an acknowledgment of all the people, beings, plant friends, and ecosystems that our lives depend on. It helps us to be more present to the world and is a support of mudita. Melody Beattie writes, "Gratitude unlocks the fullness of life. It turns what we have into enough, and more. It turns denial into acceptance, chaos into order, confusion into clarity. It can turn a meal into a feast, a house into a home, a stranger into a friend."[12]

Gratitude is not a pushing away or an ignoring of pain, but is rather holding a balance, seeing the ten thousand joys and ten thousand sorrows. Gratitude creates a tenderness of heart and therefore a container to hold the sorrows and cruelties of the world. Our practice allows us to be happy in spite of our difficulties. Even in a wounded state, the earth feeds us. Robin Wall Kimmerer writes in *Braiding Sweetgrass*, "I choose joy over despair. Not because I have my head in the sand, but because joy is what the earth gives me daily and I must return the gift."[13] It is our sacred task to find gratitude for the entirety of this human experience: the mess and the clarity, the friends and the enemies, the highs and the lows. Gratitude sustains us through difficulty. We can always find gratitude for something, as long as we are alive.

Regardless of the details of our lives, just the opportunity to live is a miracle. I remember this each time a friend has a baby. Any baby is a miracle, but in considering all of the queer parents that I know, I am familiar with all of the scheduling, effort, and money often involved in bringing queer spawn into the world. So much had to come together for each baby to emerge.

I am grateful that I chose to carry and give birth. As a trans person, my relationship to this body can be complicated. I had the necessary infrastructure to carry and birth a child, and Lezlie and I decided I would be the one to carry. I called my pregnancy "germination," which resonated as an ungendered term and one that I could relate to through my study of herbalism and farming. Germination went smoothly overall, and I know that it could have been otherwise, so I am grateful.

My labor began at three in the morning as a blizzard swirled outside, and at six o'clock I called our doula. It was amazing to witness my body do what it needed to do. I didn't have to think or exert effort necessarily, my body just went through contractions and began pushing when the time was right. I just had to let it happen. The midwife and her assistant showed up at our house and began filling the birthing tub, but baby had no patience for that. At 9:21 a.m., after six hours of active labor, squatting upon a birthing stool in our bedroom, I pushed Giuseppi's head out, then his shoulders, and then the gooey blob of baby all emerged. He cried immediately, and my partner and I held him between our two naked chests, looking at each other and him again and again, surprised despite years of planning. We had a baby in our arms! The sun emerged, gleaming off the fresh snow and brightening the room, and our little family was in bed, being served coconut rice, salmon, and berries by our beloved doula.

I could have chosen to bring a child into our lives in another way, and yet every day I am so grateful to have had this experience of childbirth. I was more embodied than I ever had been, which, as a trans person and a yogi, is saying a lot! I was prepared for that moment, to trust my body, my partner, Giuseppi, and the birth team. Through this experience, I am connected to all the other people throughout history and all over the world who have given birth, a fellowship of birthing people. I am grateful to now be a parent and connect on those grounds with so many people and creatures around the world.

Through my practice I have also learned how to have gratitude for the hard stuff—the difficult people, the US Supreme Court nominations that make me cringe, the deaths of community members and friends. All of the difficulties of my life make me who I am, have taught me about integrity, compassion, diligence, and I may not have learned the lessons otherwise. I wouldn't have chosen the difficulties, necessarily, but I wouldn't give them back, either.

My dad died when I was almost seven, two days after his own birthday. He was sixty-seven and lived what was to him a joyful life, and he knew that he risked longevity because of it. My dad was a stay-at-home dad, a kind, tender man with creases in his face from smiling. He adored me. I was incredibly connected to him, and when he died, I remained connected to his spirit, feeling him watching after me, feeling his presence at various moments of my life. My mom and dad did not raise me within any religion—I've gone to church less than ten times in my life—but his death ignited my spiritual life. I was connected to something no one else could see, a being that helped me feel safe and beloved, and that experience opened doorways to further spiritual inquiry.

At the tender age of six, a parent dying was the worst thing that could have happened to me. Malcolm Gladwell has written about the resilience of kids who lose a parent early, that that early experience creates a strength and courage carried throughout our lives. Although I grieve my dad's death, I am grateful for my spiritual life and the resilience that emerged as a result. I am grateful for his life that took a chance on love at age fifty, divorced when a no-fault divorce was legal in only few states, and began parenting again at age sixty, when he didn't have much to prove and could be a fully devoted dad. I am grateful that I have always known that I am loved, aware of what a precious thing that is.

Maya Angelou invites us, "Let gratitude be the pillow upon which you kneel to say your nightly prayer."[14] Importantly, Robin Wall Kimmerer reminds us that gratitude is reciprocal: we have a duty to protect the integrity and well-being of anything for which we are grateful.[15] Gratitude is not sentimental, it is not inconsequential, and it involves responsibility and commitment. May our gratitude for what is precious and important in this world inspire our thoughts, words, and actions.

Oppression Masquerading as Gratitude

Sometimes ableism, racism, homophobia, or other systems of oppression can masquerade as gratitude. In our aspiration of embracing all beings— those who hear and those who are deaf, those who see and those who are blind, those who walk and those who roll—we commit to value and respect all manifestations of humanity. Thus, to offer gratitude for being able to see or hear, for being able to walk and not having to roll, is a separation from and condescension toward disabled people.

A common form of oppression I see show up in both students and teachers, intended as gratitude, takes the form of "at least I'm not ___." At least I'm not incarcerated. At least I'm not in a foreign land, unable to speak the language. At least I'm not gay. Perhaps in there could be resurrected compassion for those human experiences, for there is a recognition that there is pain in that experience. However, the pain in that experience is oppression, not the experience itself. If our world were not ableist, it wouldn't be hard for disabled people to be disabled! If our world didn't target Black and Brown bodies and communities through a myriad of institutions, being Black or Brown would be just another skin color. If our world weren't homophobic, few queer folks would take their own lives or be killed at such alarming rates.

It is pity, not compassion, if there is a separation or dehumanization in a slight or grand way, which there is when one is grateful to not be X. There is a simplification of that experience, seeing the difficult struggles but not seeing the beauty, creativity, courage, brilliance, and resilience of oppressed people and communities. Many spiritual leaders have a depth of practice due to their struggle and diligent work to heal the wound and learn from it. Saint Thomas Aquinas declared that no one becomes compassionate without suffering.

We could be setting ourselves up for suffering if we orient our gratitude in such a way, for those of us who are nondisabled now are only temporarily so—all human bodies break down and succumb to injury, illness, and death eventually, as the Buddha stated. I will be disabled in the future, so how do I prepare my heart for that experience by seeing the wholeness of disabled people now, as well as the incessant reality of ableism that intersects with other aspects of identity as well? If I love disabled people now, I set myself up to love my disabled future self.

Similarly, I wonder if it's possible to not reinforce white privilege, male privilege, straight privilege, or nondisabled privilege through our gratitude practice. It is easy to reinforce it, as it is the air we breathe. If I were to say, "I'm grateful that I'm white and not a person of color," I would ask myself, why? What I'd be saying here is that I'm grateful for the system that protects me from harm by my very skin color and harms so many people due to the social construction of race. Indeed, I am not grateful for that system, for as many scholars have documented, systems of oppression dehumanize all of us—both the privileged and the oppressed. For the privileged, there's a short-term gain for a long-term loss. As a white anti-racist, I know what I have lost in my ancestors' assimilation into whiteness and white privilege. I've lost the foods, prayers, songs, wisdom, values, spiritual practices, and artistry of my people. Because of that loss and disintegration, I've turned to other cultures and traditions, such as yoga and Buddhism, as many white folks have. That then gets complicated and runs the risk of further harm through cultural appropriation. What I am wary of is ways in which we can use these practices to reinforce, rather than disrupt, systems of oppression. These practices are a tool, and like any other tool, they can be used to heal or harm.

It is different to be grateful for an aspect of my identity that doesn't grant me privilege, like my queerness. I'm not benefitted by society for being queer. Queer folks and queer culture are awesome, and I am grateful for our ways of being in the world. Gratitude toward targeted aspects of our identities is a practice of resilient self-love in a culture constantly on the attack. For targeted peoples, self-love is imperative to survival. More on that in the next chapter.

Generosity

Generosity invites us to be alert to all of the many opportunities in which to care for others. There is a freedom in generosity, a recognition of not needing, of having enough, regardless of "how much" one actually has.

According to the Buddha, generosity is a central tenet of spiritual life. Generosity is the first of the ten *paramitas* in Theravadan Buddhism, or perfections of the heart, and it is the first practice given to laypeople—to give time, energy, attention, and resources to others. When I give of time, attention, or resources, that sharing reminds me of what I do have—in the sharing is a recognition of enoughness.

Generosity involves letting go, caring for others, and a recognition of our interdependence. We let go of what we have, which is a practice in itself. We direct what we let go of toward those who may benefit, and we recognize that when those around us do better, we all do better. The Buddha spoke of generosity as benefitting your own heart three times: you gladden your heart when you are thinking of something to give, you take joy in the actual delivery, and when you remember what you gave it lifts your spirits. Every spiritual tradition that I know of has a tradition of service, of helping out. This is both community building and also self-serving, for it gets you out of your own drama and expands your perspective.

Meditation retreats that I have attended operate by *dana,* or generosity. We pay for room and board up front, but the teachers are not paid and instead are offered dana at the close of a retreat. This is a way to make the teachings accessible and for the payment to be part of one's practice. In each retreat, a dana talk is given at the end, in which the teacher or community member offers up their own practice of dana, and each time I listen, wide open from days of retreat, my own practice deepens. This practice of dana has grown to influence many areas of my life, to remind me that I can both receive and give in any exchange as a spiritual practice. In a retreat I sat with Sharon Salzberg, she suggested in our practice of generosity that when you think of giving, actually follow through. Many of us might often think of a card to send, a gift to offer, or support to put forth, but making it happen is another thing. Sharon suggested that doubt arises when we allow the impulse toward generosity just to sit—so act on it!

I have committed to giving away 10 percent of my income. Running my own business teaching yoga and dharma, sometimes I do well and some months I really struggle. Each year when I do my taxes, I go over all of my donations. It allows me to review the last year and remember, with a hand over my heart—*oh gosh, that earthquake or hurricane that devastated this group of people,* or *oh yes, the momentum of that campaign,* or *wow, that trans person has had surgery now!* I remember all of the movements I care about and am dedicated to; I remember those in my communities who struggled or succeeded. Consistently dedicating this portion of my income has made doing taxes fun due to my practice of generosity.

One of my practices during the 2020 pandemic was to send out weekly newsletters about the theme of my classes that week, and as an invitation and reminder to my students to practice. Each week in the newsletter I highlighted some of the organizations doing work that was politically relevant in the moment: organizations supporting frontline workers at meatpacking plants, funds for undocumented domestic workers and farm workers to replace the stimulus checks that documented immigrants and citizens received, Black Visions Collective when George Floyd was killed, legal organizations defending families that had been split apart at the border or deported, organizations doing get-out-the-vote work in the fall. Each week in putting together the newsletter, I would reach out to grass-roots organizer friends for recommendations of organizations. Each week I would post a piece of the organization's mission as well as why I valued the organization, and I would make my own donation. I learned about so many organizations doing such good work, and new campaigns among familiar organizations! It was such joy to do this research, and it gave me hope in a time of desperation, disregard by the federal government, and uncertainty.

True happiness is not dependent on life always being pleasurable or fun. True happiness comes from living in harmony with the ten thousand joys and the ten thousand sorrows of life. This means we can be happy in the midst of our pain. When our hearts learn to meet pain with compassion and meet pleasure with unattached appreciation, happiness can coexist with any sensation, emotion, or experience.

Among the benefits of *metta,* lovingkindness, the Buddha said, are that we sleep easily, that we awaken contented, and that when we die we have no regrets. Jack Kornfield teaches about the questions we hold in our final moments: Did I love well? Did I live fully? Did I learn to let go? The practice of mudita is one of living fully, celebrating the good, and enjoying this life that was given to us with gratitude, such that, like Zen teacher Maureen Stuart is reported to have said, we can just say thank you on our way out, without grievance or dissatisfaction.

PRACTICE: MEDITATION ON SYMPATHETIC JOY

Find a comfortable posture, sitting in a chair, upon a cushion, or even standing. Become aware of the joys, delights, and pleasures in your life recently. Remind yourself that you are deserving of joy, like everyone else. Holding your joys in your awareness, offer the following phrase:

May I be present to, and fully take in my joy.

May my joy and success continue and grow.

Now consider someone whom it is relatively easy to rejoice for, and actively recognize whatever joy or success is present in their lives. Working for some minutes with this person, picturing them in your mind's eye, begin to silently offer this person the same phrase:

May I be present to, and fully take in your joy.

May your joy and success continue and grow.

Continue to offer these words for several minutes, and then draw your attention back to your own heart, to check in and notice what has arisen.

Following this, begin to offer mudita to a neutral person. Next, offer mudita to a difficult person. Finally, offer mudita to someone who has a lot of success and pleasure. Over time this will diminish the tendencies of the mind toward comparison, jealousy, and judgment.

LOVING OURSELVES
WHOLE

The soul has no gender.
—JAYA DEVI BHAGAVATI

We are so much more than what meets the eye.
—LARRY YANG

LOVINGKINDNESS, OR *METTA* in Pali and *maitri* in Sanskrit, is the
bold practice of unconditionally welcoming our whole selves and all beings
into our hearts. It is the first practice of the Brahma Viharas in Buddhism
and is considered an umbrella practice of unconditionally and relentlessly
offering love. Metta is a fierce practice that the Buddha taught when his
monks were afraid to meditate in the forest because of forest spirits. Metta
is a cloak of protection and an invitation to put down armor, asserting that
everyone is deserving of love, just by being, just by existing; there is nothing to do to prove ourselves "worthy." We are already lovable, as is. This is a
transformative practice that uproots all the lies and judgments we've been
taught about ourselves, however we've internalized oppression, and everything we've come to believe about one another. Whoever we are, whatever
our lived experience, whatever we've done or not done, we each deserve love.

Regularly practicing lovingkindness activates and strengthens areas of the brain that are responsible for empathy and emotional intelligence, literally restructuring the brain and making the neural pathways of patience, care, focus, and wisdom stronger over time. The scientific findings about practice are important and verify what the Buddha knew millennia ago, and what practitioners since have confirmed and reconfirmed—that meditation transforms the brain to be kinder, to respond more skillfully over time. This provides further inspiration for practice—when we meditate with metta we are resculpting our brains to be brains that are compassionate in a moment of pain, that celebrate joy but know that it is fleeting, that greet others as friends rather than foes. Meditation is the laboratory for this to happen; how we live each moment off of the mat or cushion is the application of our practice. At the end of a retreat once, Larry Yang said, "And now, on to the retreat of your lives!"

We are invited to know our Buddha nature, our basic goodness, and work to see that in everyone around us. We may have to look quite diligently to find the goodness in some people! Sometimes it's also quite difficult to see it in myself, when I'm caught in a spiral of self-doubt or low self-esteem. When I can't see someone else's goodness, I am often disconnected from my own.

In metta practice, we open our hearts to the humans who share our life experience, and those who do not. We open our hearts to those above and below, the seen and the unseen, the near and the far away, the born and the yet to be born. Every being has a Buddha nature. Every one of us is basically good. Can you treat everyone around you *as* the Buddha? As you might treat the Buddha if you met him? Or as how you imagine an awakened being would treat you? And if you cannot do that, why not? Why can I not be friendly toward this person?

My colleague Molly Lannon Kenny, founder of the Samarya Center, a now-closed Seattle yoga studio, said to me once, "In my fifteen years running the Samarya Center it was always our intention that every single person who came through our space felt like they were the most supremely invited guest." What a beautiful collective practice, to figure out how to deeply welcome and cherish everyone. The Samarya Center made the first deck of yoga asana cards that I had ever seen that included fat bodies, queer bodies, and people of color—it was a breath of fresh air. That yoga deck arose out of their spiritual practice to honor everyone—to see and celebrate all bodies.

Through our practice we cultivate awareness of which habits and behaviors are wholesome seeds to water within ourselves and which are unwholesome seeds to abandon—"wholesome" meaning that which leads to connection, healing, and harmony, and "unwholesome" meaning that which is harmful or creates separation and disharmony. We are invited to learn to notice how those seeds sprout up in our lives. Who do you say hello to and who do you avoid? Who do you notice and who do you not? Who do you consider "worthy" of your attention and who is not?

Through metta, we learn to love ourselves and we learn to love others around us, and we don't sacrifice one for another but rather work to balance self-care and collective care. We begin to care about other beings around us, from our loved ones to "strangers" to difficult people, not for their benefit but because we are individually healthier and happier when we have this attitude of friendliness. It benefits others but it's not altruistic; it is rather quite self-serving. The Dalai Lama teaches that when we are only invested in our own happiness, we are invested in the happiness of one single being, and loving that one person certainly benefits us personally. But when we are invested in the happiness of all other beings on the planet, that happiness increases by billions! So-called neutral people who have neither a positive nor a negative impact on our life, who we may see in the grocery store, walking down the street, or what have you, begin to enter our sphere of awareness. Eric Kolvig describes having a practice of working to befriend everyone and treating everyone around him as his personal friend. He reports from this practice that people respond to love; it is wired within us. He even tries to love those who put up a great deal of resistance, taking it as a personal challenge to befriend *everyone*.

Metta, Privilege, and Oppression

There is a profound relationship between our personal practice and our collective experience, Larry Yang teaches. A connection exists between our internal and societal transformation. What we do in our practice is not just an internal experience. Our practice invites us to study the root of our behavior and whether it comes from love or fear. The soul has no gender, no race, no age, but is simultaneously richer for the particulars of our individual experience through race, age, gender, dis/ability, and other signifiers. We need spiritual communities to acknowledge each particular experience as part of the oneness or commonality of humanity. To go to oneness without recognizing the impact that oppression and privilege has on each of our experiences is called a spiritual bypass, a term coined by Buddhist teacher John Welwood.

Privilege has a lot to do with the spiritual bypass, because for some of us, or for some pieces of our experience, it is written into the fabric of our society as "the norm," even within our sanghas and spiritual communities. It can be easy to disregard other experiences or move toward the idea of oneness because our experience has been affirmed all along. It is painful to look at the reality of hierarchy, separation, and suffering due to the rewarding of certain embodied experiences over others. Yet we must, if we are to recognize our full humanity or to see the full humanity of any other being. As a white person, because of structural racism I don't have to look at racism as part of my daily reality, but if I don't examine it I cut off a part of myself and certainly cut myself off from a majority of the world. Francis Weller, in discussing grief on a collective level, says, "We have not reconciled with the indigenous people of this country or the people we brought here from Africa. That grief is still there in our collective psyche. We've barely touched it."[1] To realize it and speak about it is to move toward and through the pain of it and access a deeper experience and understanding on the other side.

Many of us, due to marginalized identities, must look at oppression every single day because it is on our doorsteps, in our food, in the air we breathe, constructs our physical environment, and is inherited from our ancestors. At the same time, those in power deny, dismiss, resist, or avoid marginalized experiences and histories because it's inconvenient to reckon with, painful to witness, or confusing to their worldview. This can create both a deep wound and an attachment to our experience because it's painful in the first place, and then we have to fight for acknowledgment and recognition. This can be destabilizing and disorienting because we have this experience and then are told it's not true, that it's not so bad, and that it's our own fault.

Eric Kolvig reflects, after years of work in the movement to end childhood sexual abuse, "The way that abuse is perpetuated through generations, is that the adults in the child's life can't know and are in denial, that it is too disruptive to do something."[2] Similarly, when white people can't acknowledge the impact of slavery, Jim Crow policies, racist immigration policies, and the genocide of Native people, which all led to the wealth and power of the United States, then the violence of racism is perpetuated. We have to examine our particular experience and open ourselves up to the experiences of others that are vastly different from our own in order for healing to occur. In healing these oppressions, we give ourselves the opportunity to really see our true selves.

It is no wonder that those of us with marginalized identities respond to this trauma of perpetual dismissal, disregard, pain, blame, and shame with either an attachment and holding fast to our identities—reluctant to go toward oneness out of fear of erasure, assimilation, or death—or an avoidance of the pain and a desire to go directly to oneness, recycling the idea that we too don't see race or other human differences. This is any human being's instinctive reaction to pain manifested on a societal level. If we individually don't have a practice of moving toward, investigating, and healing pain, then our society will not either.

In her poem "For the White Person Who Wants to Know How to Be My Friend," Pat Parker wrote, "The first thing you do is to forget that i'm Black. / Second, you must never forget that i'm Black."[3] We need both to be recognized for our individual experience, and for our basic humanity to be seen and recognized, regardless of our embodiment or history. If we don't recognize the particulars of our experience and the ways that they differ between each human being, as well as the patterns among various communities, that is a spiritual bypass. Larry Yang says, "We have to notice the particular on the way to the universal," for otherwise the particular experiences of a small percentage of people (white, cisgender, male, nondisabled, young, and wealthy) on the planet are mapped onto all beings, and in that we lose so much richness and bypass so much suffering. This does not make the suffering and injustice go away, but rather more deeply ingrains it.

In marginalized communities we can run the risk of becoming attached to our identities and seeing how we are received in the world as who we *really are*. At the same time, any marginalized community has a well of incredible strength, courage, resilience, and spiritual depth because individual and collective survival depends on it. In this experience, we know, feel, and breathe our spiritual potential and our sense of oneness, but we cannot collectively arrive without a recognition of the particular realities of each of our experience, which is layered in identity. We do have so much more in common than what separates us.

Any marginalized position in society is an experience that is not recognized, portrayed, or centered. Our movements fight for this; we fight for our needs to be seen and recognized, for our experiences to be portrayed, and for our needs to be centered. At some point along the way, we need to loosen and let go of our identities as being the whole of who we are. The teachings tell us that attachment creates suffering, Larry Yang tells us that we are so much more than what meets the eye, and Jaya Devi teaches that the soul has no gender. So what if your beauty lies both within *and* beyond your Blackness? If my beauty lies within and beyond my queerness? There is a balance between loving ourselves within our identity and being attached to the identity.

Concurrently, within some social justice circles, in the effort to center those most marginalized and out of an unexamined reaction to systems of oppression, we may inadvertently or intentionally devalue or dismiss the pain of people with privilege. I have worked with white folks, men, and straight folks embedded in social justice to love themselves as well. This is important—our activism has to come out of a holistic metta, for those most targeted by systems of power and for those most protected. Jaya Devi's guru, Ma Jaya, said that "pain is pain." Regardless of whose it is, pain matters, and we must tend to it and heal it; if we don't tend to it with attention and care, out of that pain grows rage, aggression, addiction, resentment, and fear. We see untended pain and trauma in current white supremacist movements; in a white anti-racist group I'm a part of, a friend said, "What if we really *do* have to care about white men's pain?" We have seen what can happen if that pain is not tended to. Perhaps as a fellow white person I must tend to white men's pain; that may be a corner of the racial justice movement for me. When I can tend to their pain, perhaps they don't act out on my friends and siblings of color. Our identities influence how we are regarded and treated in this world, *and* we are so much more than what meets the eye.

If I exclude or push anyone away, my heart is not free. When we push someone out of our hearts there is a contraction, whether we feel superior or inferior in a hierarchy or condemn ourselves in the relationship. Our practice of metta is influenced by what we've inherited in our world—racism, classism, sexism, transphobia, ableism, homophobia—whether we've been harmed or protected by these systems. We begin with working deep within our hearts, and then having our words and actions match our greatest intention to welcome everyone into our hearts. When we aspire to have the eyes of a bodhisattva, to look upon all beings with love and compassion, as a community and individually, it inevitably shifts how we show up in community.

Sharon Salzberg tells a story of her experience in working with metta:

After I had spent these six weeks doing the metta meditation all day long, my teacher, U Pandita, called me into his room and said, "Say you were walking in the forest with your benefactor, your friend, your neutral person, and your enemy. Bandits come up and demand that you choose one person in your group to be sacrificed. Which one would you choose to die?"

I was shocked at U Pandita's question. I sat there and looked deep into my heart, trying to find a basis from which I could choose. I saw that I could not feel any distinction between any of those people, including myself. Finally I looked at U Pandita and replied, "I couldn't choose; everyone seems the same to me."

U Pandita then asked, "You wouldn't choose your enemy?" I thought a minute and then answered, "No, I couldn't."

Finally U Pandita asked me, "Don't you think you should be able to sacrifice yourself to save the others?" He asked the question as if more than anything else in the world he wanted me to say, "Yes, I'd sacrifice myself." A lot of conditioning rose up in me—an urge to please him, to be "right" and to win approval. But there was no way I could honestly say "yes," so I said, "No, I can't see any difference between myself and any of the others." He simply nodded in response, and I left.[4]

In relationships with colleagues, when I am deliberately working across race, class, and sexual orientation differences, inevitably the systems of oppression arise. It is par for the course. My practice of equanimity teaches me to take the larger view, the larger perspective, rather than getting caught in the drama of the moment, considering, "Who is this work serving? What might happen in the future if we build this relationship?" And my practice of metta encourages me to plant seeds of love, which will overcome the many seeds of hate that have been planted and cultivated for centuries. I have come to expect that dynamics of oppression and privilege will arise in any relationship, and to trust that my practice can hold them. They may break a relationship or make it stronger; it depends. Systems of oppression are dismantled through relationships, forgiveness, accountability, and leveraging privilege for the benefit of all. If I can hold that intention in my heart through the difficult conversations regarding my own words or actions that uphold white supremacy, transphobia, and ableism and that harm myself and my family daily, and slow down and listen when a wound of mine or a coworker's is scratched, I can grow my heart wider and be in integrity.

Metta has been one of the most transformative practices in my life, and I've seen evidence because my relationships have improved over time. One of the original co-owners of Third Root once commented on how I have become kinder over the years. In my relationships, how and what is communicated, how authentic and real we each can be, and the ways that we show up to support or allow in support has shifted. I've also seen a shift in which relationships take more of a center stage (those that are more loving, honest, and mutual) and which have fallen away (those that are more superficial, based on gossip, or one-sided in efforts to maintain the relationship). My intimate partnership has improved and relationships with my family, relationships with colleagues, and the ways in which I interact with rude "strangers" (or even seeing them as "strangers" at all) have become more skillful, as have the ways I care for myself. I enjoy my life more and feel more connected.

The practice of metta involves faith: faith that this practice makes a difference for us and in the world. At the end of many classes and retreats, we send out metta to all beings, or dedicate the merit to either specific communities that are in the midst of difficulty or to ourselves. Sometimes this can feel trite or sentimental. Other times it can feel mechanical. The laws of karma dictate that the energy that we put out there is the energy that comes back to us, yet its timing is capricious and undetermined. We are entitled to our actions, but not the fruit of our actions. Our actions will inevitably have some effect—protecting us, resculpting our own brains, creating friendships and connection, and healing where harm has occurred—but the effect is out of our control.

Loving Ourselves

Loving ourselves is deep work, and as I teach lovingkindness workshops I find that whether I am teaching in an elite, expensive yoga studio or a maximum security prison, the most difficult work for my students is in offering love and kindness to themselves as individuals, for we have been taught self-hatred in the interest of capitalism. If we believe that we aren't lovable, that we are disposable, that we are not capable of great things, when we bring that into our hearts and souls, we do the powers that be a great favor. Steve Biko, a great anti-apartheid organizer in South Africa, said, "The most potent weapon in the hands of the oppressors is the mind of the oppressed."[5] Self-love, then, is an effective tool of liberation.

In the essay "They Can't Turn Back," James Baldwin reflected, "It took many years of vomiting up all the filth that I had been taught about myself and had believed before I could walk on the earth as if I had a right to be."[6] You cannot live in this culture and not be conditioned by the myths of who is a valuable, important human and who is disposable, an inconvenience, an embarrassment. The exciting news is that through practice, we have the capacity to shift those beliefs, and potentially avoid passing them on to the next generations.

In her 2001 show *Notorious C.H.O.*, Margaret Cho said,

If you are a woman, if you're a person of color, if you are gay, lesbian, bisexual, transgender, if you are a person of size, if you are a person of intelligence, if you are a person of integrity, then you are considered a minority in this world. You know when you look in the mirror and you think "oh, I'm so fat,

I'm so old, I'm so ugly," don't you know, that's not your authentic self? But that is billions upon billions of dollars of advertising, magazines, movies, billboards, all geared to make you feel shitty about yourself so that you will take your hard-earned money and spend it at the mall on some turn-around creme that doesn't turn around shit. When you don't have self-esteem you will hesitate before you do anything in your life. You will hesitate to go for the job you really wanna go for, you will hesitate to ask for a raise, you will hesitate to call yourself an American, you will hesitate to report a rape, you will hesitate to defend yourself when you are discriminated against because of your race, your sexuality, your size, your gender. You will hesitate to vote, you will hesitate to dream. For us to have self-esteem is truly an act of revolution and our revolution is long overdue.[7]

Honoring that we are so much more than meets the eyes, for ourselves, is a radical act because it claims our humanity, it asserts our spiritual essence, it declares our right to be on this earth and be greeted gently and respectfully, for every one of us. Audre Lorde, in her poem "A Litany for Survival," says, "We were never meant to survive."[8] Any marginalized people, in our fullest sense, were not meant to survive—the system was built on our disposability and destruction.

Many of us, due to oppression, are taught that we are not enough, that we are not lovable as we are. Fat people, people of color, disabled people, trans people, queer folks, rural people, working-class people, undocumented people—we are constantly faced with this message in the world, which is the insidious nature of oppression. Being ourselves, and loving ourselves, is difficult when the whole world around us is telling us that we are unacceptable and unlovable, when we see our friends, comrades, and lovers either killed or take their own lives, overwhelmed by the struggle of continuing to live. It is a political act to keep ourselves alive, to love ourselves as we are, and to work toward loving all of humanity in all of its various expressions, resisting the internalization of the message that anyone is at their core unlovable.

Laverne Cox said on her Tumblr blog after Caitlyn Jenner came out as trans,

It feels like a new day, indeed, when a trans person can present her authentic self to the world for the first time and be celebrated for it so universally. Many

have commented on how gorgeous Caitlyn looks in her photos, how she is "slaying for the Gods." I must echo these comments in the vernacular, "Yasss Gawd! Werk Caitlyn! Get it!" But this has made me reflect critically on my own desires to "work a photo shoot," to serve up various forms of glamour, power, sexiness, body affirming, racially empowering images of the various sides of my black, trans womanhood. I love working a photo shoot and creating inspiring images for my fans, for the world and above all for myself. But I also hope that it is my talent, my intelligence, my heart and spirit that most captivate, inspire, move and encourage folks to think more critically about the world around them. Yes, Caitlyn looks amazing and is beautiful but what I think is most beautiful about her is her heart and soul, the ways she has allowed the world into her vulnerabilities. The love and devotion she has for her family and that they have for her. Her courage to move past denial into her truth so publicly. These things are beyond beautiful to me. A year ago when my Time *magazine cover came out I saw posts from many trans folks saying that I am "drop dead gorgeous" and that that doesn't represent most trans people. (It was news to [me] that I am drop dead gorgeous but I'll certainly take it). But what I think they meant is that in certain lighting, at certain angles I am able to embody certain cisnormative beauty standards. Now, there are many trans folks because of genetics and/or lack of material access who will never be able to embody these standards. More importantly many trans folks don't want to embody them and we shouldn't have to to be seen as ourselves and respected as ourselves. It is important to note that these standards are also informed by race, class and ability among other intersections. I have always been aware that I can never represent all trans people. No one or two or three trans people can. This is why we need diverse media representations of trans folks to multiply trans narratives in the media and depict our beautiful diversities. I started #TransIsBeautiful as a way to celebrate all those things that make trans folks uniquely trans, those things that don't necessarily align with cisnormative beauty standards. For me it is necessary everyday to celebrate every aspect of myself especially those things about myself that don't align with other people's ideas about what is beautiful. #TransIsBeautiful is about, whether you're trans or not, celebrating all those things that make us uniquely ourselves.[9]*

Laverne Cox invites us to cultivate love, for ourselves and others, rather than reproduce and perpetrate violence. I cherish the way that Buddhism contributes to my perspective on social justice, that through each thought, word, and deed we can create love, healing, and justice or we can pass on injustice, pain, and violence. Every single thing I do and every single word I utter matters.

Melody Moore is a colleague who heads the organization Embody Love Movement, working with girls and women around body image. Melody has a history of distorted body image and came from a family where her value had a lot to do with her appearance. Professionally, Melody began to specialize in working with people with eating disorders and distorted body image. In a workshop with Melody, I was struck when she said that she has stopped checking herself out in the mirror—critiquing her belly, scrutinizing her appearance—because she realized that it was a subtle form of violence against herself. It reminded me of Margaret Cho's quote, and I thought that Melody was completing the thought—that yes, we need to develop self-esteem and boost that of others, and we also must notice where we are putting our energy and consider whether it is contributing to our vitality, creativity, and sense of connection to ourselves and others or whether it's detracting from it. Melody then shared that now it is her practice, when she has the inkling to check herself out in the mirror, to get closer to the mirror, and look deep into her own eyes, because that is where her beauty lies. She takes this moment of potential self-harm and turns it into self-love, and these small acts add up, over time, to really loving herself.

Loving ourselves exactly as we are—meeting beauty standards or not, being "productive citizens" or not—is hard work. Self-love is so incredibly important in living whole, healthy lives, having strong relationships and meaningful work, and a slew of other implications, as Margaret Cho notes. Through metta we are invited to examine the ways in which we care for ourselves, to get curious about our inner self-talk and contemplate our relationships as nourishing and enlivening or depleting and draining. This is not to say that we shy away from the hard work of relationships, especially close ones, but that out of our self-love we discern which relationships are leading toward growth and which unnecessarily suck our life force out. In offering metta to ourselves, we confront the messages the world has fed us and that we have eaten up, and we come to know ourselves as inherently deserving of love, kindness, and respect, just like everyone else.

Warming the Heart by Loving Benefactors

The second category of people that we work within the Brahma Viharas are called benefactors. These are people with whom we have only a positive relationship, people who have guided us, people who we look up to or admire. A benefactor is usually not someone closer than that or where the relationship is mutual, because inevitably there is some level of conflict with some level of intimacy. There is benefit to this distance—there is a certain kind of safety and formality to the relationship.

Working with a benefactor has been a way for me to honor, in a formal and consistent way, all those who came before me—my ancestors, social justice movement ancestors, queer ancestors. These are people who don't know me, necessarily. They may never know me. But just by their being alive, or having been alive, I benefit from them.

The person who most consistently occupies this category for me is Toni Morrison. I know people who knew her, but I never saw her in person and certainly never met her. I've read most of her books and read much commentary, especially from Black feminists, about her books and their benefit to Black lives. When I offer metta to Toni Morrison, I am bowing to her, saluting her, holding her in reverence, continuing to learn from her about lives both quite different from and quite similar to my own. I bow to everything that held Toni Morrison up, all the conditions that supported her in her writing, mentorship, and leadership.

On a few occasions, I have resumed contact with a person in the category of benefactor—a mentor and a teacher with whom I had fallen out of contact with—which shifted the individual from the category of benefactor. What I learned from these experiences is that sometimes it's fine to allow a teacher in the past to remain a teacher in the past, having served a particular purpose at a particular moment. In both situations, meeting them again when I was at a different age, a different point in my practice, changed the relationship.

As a teacher in my college years, Lillian was marvelous. She was my first yoga teacher, and I became a member of her Sunday 8:00 a.m. Zen sangha during my junior and senior years of college. The sangha included a poetry professor, a university administrator, a local woodworker, and some other folks, and it connected me with people living their lives outside of the campus bubble, which gave me perspective and grounding with regards to my college experience. When I contacted Lillian years later, she asked about my "sex change" and conveyed some of her own ignorance and transphobia, which shifted her out of the category of benefactor! The relationship was no longer solely positive.

I met Cynthia during a summer when I was in college and wanted to live and work in Alaska. She worked for the American Friends Service Committee and involved me in her work on subsistence, a hot topic in Alaska. She ran a "listening project" where people from different corners of the conflict met to hear each other's experience and connect with one another's hearts before moving forward with policies. This profoundly impacted my social justice work, joining together spiritual practice with political change. When I visited Cynthia years later, our connection was no longer as potent and compelling; she was no longer in the role of mentor and I wasn't looking for guidance and support in the same way.

On stormy days, working with a benefactor reminds me of my heart's capacity to love. When this heart is sore, reluctant, and cranky, sometimes I only work with the benefactor in metta meditation. This is the purpose of this category of benefactor—it primes the heart for the other work of metta, reminds us of what is possible with people in other categories. Offering metta to someone easy to love, respect, and admire strengthens the heart and prepares us for loving those who are more difficult or complicated.

Expanding Circles of Care by Loving Neutral People

Another category of people we are invited to turn toward is "neutral people." These are people who are familiar or recognizable, but you don't know the details of their lives—what has brought them sorrow or joy. You may not even know their names. They have a neutral impact on your life. This works against the wiring of our nervous systems that responds to neutral stimuli with indifference. In offering metta toward a neutral person, we rewire and pay attention.

Sharon Salzberg tells this story of the health benefits of developing a loving heart:

> *Researchers once gave a plant to every resident of a nursing home. They told half of these elderly people that the plants were theirs to care for — they had to pay close attention to their plants' needs for water and sunlight, and they had to respond carefully to those needs. The researchers told the other half of the residents that their plants were theirs to enjoy but that they did not have to take any responsibility for them; the nursing staff would care for the plants.*
>
> *At the end of a year, the researchers compared the two groups of elders. The residents who had been asked to care for their plants were living considerably longer than the norm, were much healthier, and were more oriented towards and connected to their world. The other residents, those who had plants but did not have to stay responsive to them, simply reflected the norms for people their age in longevity, health, alertness, and engagement with the world.*[10]

Offering love and care outward is good for us! There are endless opportunities. For the nursing home residents, the plants began as their neutral being. Through caring for it, the plants lived well and the residents' health improved.

What is beautiful about working with a neutral being is that just by offering metta toward this being, whose name you don't know, you can shift your relationship with them. The neutral people I've worked with have become memorable in my life. My postal clerk Alicia here in Salt Lake City, a cashier named Dawn at the natural food store, Demani the preadolescent who lived on my floor in Brooklyn with his brothers and mother, the yoga student who I see in the studio but who doesn't attend my classes, the barking dog down the street, the evasive cat that I saw in my Massachusetts neighborhood—all became my friends, even if they never knew it, due to my work with the neutral category in my practice. On the block I lived on in Flatbush, Brooklyn, there was a skinny older gentleman who drank coffee out of a blue paper cup from the bodega on the corner every morning. I would see him every morning when I walked my Rottweiler, Tulsi. Because he was a neutral person in my metta practice, I started to notice more and more about him. I asked his name; I interacted with him more and more. He became a friend.

Expanding our circles of care is important in a world so divided. Metta invites us to befriend everyone. Eric Kolvig's practice of befriending everyone, finding common ground with everyone, feeds unity and connection rather than separation and judgment. There are billions of neutral beings in the world, a potentially endless practice. The exploration here is what happens in your own heart in that process of extending lovingkindness. All of these practices have been practiced by millions of people before you, yet you are invited to try on the practice for yourself and see what resonates, what improves your life. Offering metta toward neutral people has made me a more conscientious person, moving through the world with ever more care, truly seeing each driver on the road, each fellow shopper in the grocery store, each fellow person walking their dog companion in my neighborhood. Through working with the neutral category of people, I am more connected to my world.

Amid Intimacy and Conflict: Loving Loved Ones

When we work with the category of loved ones, there already exists a lot of relationship and history, unlike with the neutral person. In these relationships there is a great deal of care and intimacy, and there has also probably been some pain and conflict. The task in offering metta to loved ones is one of letting go of stories, history, expectations, disappointments, and betrayals, and offering them lovingkindness unconditionally. We honor and connect to our beloveds' basic goodness, witnessing their wholeness and offering our love.

At times, loved ones are an incredible boon, and at other times they can rub you in the worst way. My mom, my partner, and my closest friends have all spanned the categories here of benefactor, loved one, and difficult person. Working with a loved one in metta practice brings me back to the connection present in the relationship and the many reasons that I love this person, and this gratitude enlivens the relationship. Sometimes our loved ones are easy to love, to celebrate, to care for, to support.

Sometimes, when there is conflict in a relationship, I do a metta meditation that includes just me and this other person. I offer kindness and care to myself, which sometimes allows me to recognize the ways in which I'm depleted, overwhelmed, overextended—all of which contribute to conflict in the relationship! I offer metta to the other person, reminding myself why I'm in it with them, working out being more loving to people in close proximity. This work on my cushion has been incredibly useful in resolving conflict, enabling me to see the other person's side of the conflict, their interests, and that what they bring to the conflict may arise out of something having nothing to do with me. Therefore, the conflict becomes less personal and more workable—not something wrong with me or wrong with them but rather two people, dizzied by the demands of life, knocking into each other unmindfully. I can see what we each need, how I can show up for those needs, and that the conflict, no matter how petty or grand, is workable.

Working with the category of loved ones has also served me in remaining connected to those whom I'm no longer in close proximity with. Offering metta to my friend in the Hudson Valley, whom I befriended in Ithaca, or to my niece, who I lived with in Atlanta and now lives in San Francisco with her wife and daughter, means I bring the love, care, connection, meaning, and beauty of the relationship to my heart wherever I am. It reminds me that I am never separate from those I love.

Doing the Deep Work: Loving Our Enemies

The aim of metta is to let all beings into our hearts—even those who have committed the worst atrocities against our ancestors, families, communities, or in the world at large. We trust and invest in compassion and forgiveness as part of loving the enemy. We can be change agents, returning kindness and integrity in the face of it all, passing on love and not fear, getting curious about where that path leads. The teaching of metta to love our "enemies" or difficult people in our lives involves a willingness to put down the story, to set aside our need to be right. The Buddha said that he taught two things: suffering and the end of suffering. Difficult people may have caused suffering in our life, but can we choose to heal, rather than pass on the suffering? If we recognize that "hurt people hurt people," in a deep way, then might we become invested in everyone's happiness and well-being, because it will benefit all? Jesse Amesmith, owner of YogaVibe Rochester, where I taught for a year, says, "We all do well when we all do well."

Out of concern for our own well-being, born out of love, we might practice discernment in metta. Opening your heart to someone is not the same as opening your home to someone. At what distance or proximity can you love a particular person well? For some people, it may be thousands of miles! For others, you may share a bed each night. For someone who has hurt you repeatedly, perhaps it's wise to not let them close, but to love them from a distance; that boundary is an act of love toward yourself.

Fear arises for us when we go from a place of safety to the unknown. At the same time, fear is an ally that calls on us to stretch ourselves, to grow, which is what "loving the enemy" calls on us to do.

For me, the work of loving my enemies has taken many directions, from professional work colleagues, coworkers who my lived experience has taught me are my enemies, to people who this culture has taught me to distrust or dehumanize, to people who share aspects of my own identity. I have learned that harm can happen anywhere, that I am not "safe" from harm anywhere, that there is in fact no "safe space." When I came out as trans in 2004, queer cisgender women asked the most invasive questions of me and were incredibly unwelcoming; previously, this had been my community, the community that I felt most at home in. Now, I am grateful for these women, who illuminated an important lesson for me: I can neither assume safety based on identity nor anticipate harm based on identity. I have learned that when I might assume someone to be either difficult or an ally to me based on their identities and perceived life's experience, before really knowing them, I am setting myself up for potential suffering. Yes, certain aspects of identity may mean that we share some experience or perspective of the world, but at the same time, some people may not have healed or are in a cycle of rage or grief that prevents connection.

I have learned and internalized, and now have to unlearn, that those who cause harm in the world are fundamentally different from me. This story is that they have a messed-up conception of the world or that they are so privileged as to have never experienced pain. Through activism that seeks to fight injustice and the dehumanization of marginalized people and be led by those most affected, I have learned to dehumanize those with power. Through my practice and with the guidance of teachers and mentors, I have learned to honor their humanity, to meet them there. I remind myself again that hatred does not cease through hatred. Part of my own liberation may be ceasing my own projection of separation while seeking connection in a way in which I am not attached to results. I have learned that the courage to be vulnerable with my "enemies" and difficult people, or even people who elicit distrust or fear within me, more often than not creates connection and possibility—or, in the absence of that relationship building, makes me stronger and more courageous.

A few years ago, Seane Corn was working on her submission to the anthology *Yoga and Body Image,* edited by Melanie Klein and Anna Guest-Jelley, and asked for my help. She and I had worked together for about a year or a little more at that point. Previously, I had been aware of her and her organization Off the Mat, Into the World for years, but I had been suspicious of their work and that of colleagues of mine who had been involved in various ways—skeptical of two white women and a mixed-race woman, resistant to their media images, critical of their Seva program in Haiti, Cambodia, and Uganda, which I saw as perpetuating the tradition of white women trying to "save" brown children. After meeting Seane in 2011, she pulled me in, and gave me a scholarship to attend the Off the Mat leadership development program. This began a deep relationship with the entire organization, and now I am on their faculty! As Seane was working on her submission for *Yoga and Body Image,* she asked if I could tear it to shreds, to be her harshest critic.

This was an honor for me, to contribute to a draft of Seane's submission and utilize my activist critique, examining whose experience is centered and who is excluded or disregarded. This moment was built upon other trust-building moments, as I had come to trust Seane and understand that she was on my side, that she understood my experience in the world and supported my work. In this moment, she taught me a wonderful lesson about befriending your "enemies"—that part of me that could hurt her and be overly critical could be useful to her if she drew me in, built relationship, and didn't shame that part of me. Since then, many colleagues have approached me in much the same way, asking me to point out in various situations what they may be missing or dynamics that they are not aware of; this serves the yoga service work we are doing broadly and invests in creating more space for marginalized folks. In turn, I have the opportunity to practice offering skillful feedback that trusts their basic goodness, and open doors for my colleagues rather than slamming them shut while shaming them. The experience of editing Seane's piece honored that part of myself groomed through years of activism, and ensured that Seane's piece wasn't alienating people who she intends and wants to befriend and ally with and who I care about, am in community with, and am accountable to.

I was walking my dog in western New York soon after leaving Brooklyn. She pooped, I picked it up with a bag, and put it in the nearest trash can. I heard a scream from inside a nearby house, and kept walking. Then a huge white man, twice my size, stormed after me. Over my shoulder I saw him coming and turned around, took a deep breath, and walked slowly toward him. He screamed from five feet away, "What the hell are you doing in our trash can?!" I took a breath and told him, "I put my dog's poop bag in there." He yelled, "You think we want your dog's shit? We don't want your dog's shit!" I said, "Sir, would you like me to remove it?" and he screamed, "Get it the fuck out of there!" I leaned over the deep trash can, looked for the green poop bag, and pulled it out. I asked him, "Do you need anything else?" No answer. I told him, "Okay, sir, well I hope you have a good day. I hope it improves from here." He screamed, stomping away, "I always have a good day!" As I continued on my dog walk, I said over my shoulder, "I really hope that is true." I didn't take on this man's anger. I didn't need to be right. I treated him well. Sometimes it's more complicated or nuanced, but sometimes loving our enemies is just this simple.

To love my enemies I need to be nourished within myself, and I need to do the inner work of loving them, sitting with their image in metta meditation, and planting seeds of connection and respect within myself, rather than watering the seeds of anticipated betrayal and harm. I could consider many people within the category of "enemy" or difficult people: cisgender men, whom I was raised to see as self-interested and highly sexualized; middle-class straight white women, who have been some of the people who have hurt me the deepest; social justice organizers, who can have a very cutting, personal, harsh critique and can be unforgiving of mistakes; corporations and politicians who put profit before people; or those that the media and racist culture teach me to distrust or even despise, such as housing-insecure people or addicts. I try to follow Eric Kolvig's practice of befriending, and with these difficult people, to take it as a personal challenge. In this effort, I plant seeds of love rather than seeds of fear or seeds of hate, and I remain curious about where they may lead.

PRACTICE: LOVINGKINDNESS MEDITATION

First offer these phrases to yourself, then to a benefactor, then a neutral person, then a loved one, then a difficult person, and then expand it to all beings and creatures everywhere, without exception. Alternately, you can work with just one of these categories for the entire sit. Sit for at least five minutes total and as long as you like. Work with a timer so that you're not looking at the clock.

It can also be a powerful practice to offer metta to a group or community that you are a part of (such as all men, all trans people, all survivors of violence, etc.), then a group that you are not a part of, and then all of you (both different and similar) at once to break down separation or barriers to our love inside and out.

May I/you/we be loved and loving.

May I/you/we trust my/your/our inherent belonging.

May I/you/we be safe and protected.

May I/you/we be as healthy as I/you/we can be in this moment.

May I/you/we have a lasting peace.

Part 2

QUEERING YOGA

I HAVE HAD to wade through some muck to find the goodness of yogic and Buddhist teachings. My friend Teo Drake has said, "The teachings have never failed me, but the teachers certainly have." Capitalism, white supremacy, misogyny, sexual violence, fatphobia, ableism, transphobia, the gender binary, racism, and cultural appropriation are present in yoga and Buddhism in the US and are reproduced in our studios, classes, workshops, trainings, and retreats if we are not specifically aware of their dynamics and directly working to uproot them. I have witnessed countless microaggressions of many varieties in these spaces where I and other marginalized folks come to heal. Oppressive dynamics are often denied when confronted or spiritually bypassed in the name of "oneness," despite the purported aspiration of awakening. I write about some of these dynamics and experiences here, and I also explore the organizations and bodies of work that are working to transform those dynamics—work that has become my own within yoga and dharma spaces.

The biggest challenge for this work does not occur in yoga classrooms but rather within greater mainstream yoga: to gain respect and be hired as a queer, trans, anti-racist yoga teacher. It is difficult for me and members of my community to access training that respects our experience, where we can feel safe to be out as trans or queer, where our bodies and anatomy are mindfully included, and which we can financially access. I have been devalued, excluded, dismissed, disregarded, harmed, pushed out, and pathologized by whole studios, studio owners, and teachers over the years as both a student and a teacher. I do not doubt that at least part of that exclusion is due to my trans and queer identity and the social justice politic that I bring into the space. I have raised countless issues with yoga teachers, and I have designed trainings on what *not* to say while teaching yoga, based on those experiences and similar experiences shared with me by fat yogis, disabled yogis, South Asian yogis, and other yogis of color.

Very few texts on the teachings are written by queer folks, and many of those that exist have been written in the past five years. One anthology exists by trans Buddhists, but no other text exists (that I know of) about the living teachings written by a trans person. And, as my gender studies professor partner often reminds me, the identity of a person doesn't matter as much as whether they are embedded in their community, representing that community's concerns, their politics informed and guided by that community, their words and actions accountable to that community. Thus, reading a book by someone queer- and trans-identified is not necessarily different or important in the field of yoga or dharma—what matters most is the queer politic, being embedded in trans community, the practice informed by visionary and transformative social justice movements, accountable to movements led by queer and trans people of color.

In part 2 of this book, I bring critiques and apply the practices discussed in the first part. I lift up some fabulous work happening in the field of yoga and social justice, and I name dynamics of oppression reinstated again and again in mainstream yoga. This is what it is to "queer" something: to critique, challenge, and transform toward something more radical—that is, deeply rooted in truth, love, and justice. I bow to queer comrades around the world throughout time queering their fields: dance, academia, rabbinical studies, literature, music, art, seed saving, health care, the birth world, family building, real estate and design, chemistry, neuroscience, and beyond.

NOT LIVING OUR YOGA, JUST SELLING IT: YOGA AND CAPITALISM

YOGA IS A spiritual practice, but in a capitalist economy, it's also increasingly a global business. In the United States, yoga has become part of the capitalist economy. Peace of mind sells! Releasing tension in the body can put money in the pocket! If you're not anxious or depressed, you're more productive! As yoga becomes a commodity, its teachings, origins, and history are often diluted and disrespected, aspects of yoga are taken out of context, and other components, like the ethical practices, are left behind (integrity and generosity are so inconvenient to capitalism!).

I am concerned about the selling of yoga for two reasons: the practice itself may become distorted or changed due to the commercial value of some practices and teachings over others, and many people cannot afford to practice, attend retreats, or become teachers. If we examine many manifestations of yoga on this continent, we are not living our yoga, we're just selling it. Marketers realize that yoga and Buddhism are offering something that everyone wants; it's a $27 billion industry.[1] Along with the investment in the yoga and wellness industry comes cultural appropriation, which I discuss in the next chapter—it is a byproduct of capitalism.

So, wait, what is capitalism, exactly? For a simple definition I turn to *Teen Vogue*, which has been bending more and more toward justice in the last ten years: "Capitalism is defined as an economic system in which a country's trade, industry, and profits are controlled by private companies, instead of by the people whose time and labor powers those companies," writes Kim Kelly.[2] Capitalism is the market system that prioritizes profit over the planet and its people. Anti-capitalism has been central to my activism, as capitalism is used to dehumanize and dispose of people all over the planet in the name of profit and contaminate and/or destroy ecosystems in order to make more money off of the land (such as the oil fields in the Arctic National Wildlife Refuge or the rainforests of the Amazon that have been burned to use the land for farming soybeans). Under capitalism, any practice (like yoga), any tragedy (like Hurricane Sandy), any human operating value (like fearlessness or compassion) is an opportunity to make money. Capitalism is an incredibly dehumanizing economic system, building wealth for a select few while poverty rates around the world soar, environmental destruction contaminates the air, water, food, and climate that we all depend on, and communities are pitted against one another. On her blog, adrienne maree brown says, "Capitalists are absolutely looking at how to benefit from the tragedy we are currently in—medical supplies, technology control, security, borders, data access, benefiting from an economy that crashes and has to rebuild."[3] We saw this after Hurricane Katrina when entrepreneurs rushed in to capitalize off of a broken-down city and during the 2020 pandemic when the net worth of Jeff Bezos and others among the most wealthy vastly increased; simultaneously, unemployment and evictions soared and food banks' supplies did not approach meeting the need.

Capitalism is harmful to life. Yoga in its entirety supports, enhances, and heals life. We see the clash if we consider yoga in its wholeness of philosophies and practices and its vastness of many lineages across time. The first practices of yoga are the *Yamas,* or the ethical practices that point us toward thinking, speaking, and acting toward collective liberation, rather than the allure of doing what is quick, convenient, self-serving (for now), and profit making and imagining our actions as independent of everything else. Without the ethical practices we are likely to create further harm in our world, a world that is already hurting so much. Every meaningful wisdom tradition has ethical practices for this reason—for when our practice is applied in our lives, when the difficult decision arises, when our words and actions could lead toward harm or toward healing. This misguided behavior may create short-term gain, but it will ultimately hurt the whole, which includes the person who created harm. There exists great risk, then, in separating yoga asana from the Yamas. Asanas are the postures that are an aspect of the eight limbs of yoga presented in Raja Yoga and developed more extensively at least partly due to the European influence of gymnastics. Although asana is one-eighth of the path, it's marketed as if it is the whole of yoga practice. Every teacher should teach the Yamas and every student should be familiar with them and practicing them—they are the very first practices because they prevent us from making a mess in our lives (and therefore on our mats).

The Yamas of yoga consist of the following:

1. *Ahimsa*: harmlessness or lovingkindness

2. *Satya*: truthfulness and impeccable integrity

3. *Asteya*: nonstealing, gratitude, and generosity

4. *Brahmacharya*: being wise and loving with our sexual energies specifically, recognizing their unique potency, and skillful with our energy more broadly

5. *Aparigraha*: nongreed or nonattachment

The ethical practices are incredibly important on a personal level, and they are essential to social justice. If we divorce the physical asana practice from the ethical practices, we run the risk of yoga creating harm rather than participating in social justice, and individually and collectively our spiritual practice is quite shallow, allowing yoga to be taught just to the elite, to become a "market" and an "industry" rather than a practice that includes the physical but also ethics, daily observances (called the *Niyamas*), the philosophies, the breath, and meditation. If we are not knowledgeable of yoga's roots in India, and the current and historical politics of India, we are likely out of alignment in our integrity and practice of nonviolence, carrying on neocolonialism either without realizing it or quite on purpose because it makes a profit.

The ethical practices of yoga and capitalism are fundamentally at odds. Ahimsa is a commitment to do no harm; capitalism steamrolls anything standing in its way, be it a union, environmental regulations, or trust. Satya is a commitment to integrity and truthfulness; again, capitalism will do anything for profit, tell any lies, such as the lie that yoga is for skinny white athletic women. Asteya is the commitment to not take anything that is not freely offered; capitalism is built upon the theft of labor, resources, and land. Brahmacharya is the wise use of energy, especially sexual energy, to not cause harm; how often do cisgender men in power use their sexual energy to reinforce their power and domination? The #MeToo movement brought this into the mainstream. Aparigraha is the practice of nongreed and enoughness; capitalism is built upon ever-expanding markets, where no amount of profit is ever "enough."

When I discuss the yoga industry in social settings, my friends are shocked to find out the economic dynamics of yoga, as the industry of yoga differs so greatly from the teachings of yoga. I present the realities of the business of yoga in this chapter in the hopes that students of yoga can make more informed choices and ask poignant questions when they attend yoga classes, workshops, trainings, or retreats. I want to explore yoga and capitalism so that teachers know what they're getting into (or enmeshed in!), so that we can transparently discuss financial matters with one another and potentially recognize our collective power and act in solidarity with one another. This information needs to be on the table so that we can see the industry clearly on our way to envisioning a more liberatory model of sharing yoga.

Yoga Teachers Hold On by a Thread

Despite the gargantuan industry of yoga, most teachers get paid twenty to fifty dollars per drop-in class, and many teach between eight and fifteen classes per week. Many teachers cannot survive on this income, unless they are not just good but excellent at self-promotion, networking, and perseverance. A studio's income from a single sixty- to ninety-minute class is often three to five times greater than that of the teacher.

Several payment structures exist. Gyms often pay teachers per class or per hour. Many studios pay per student, and some have a base level that they pay teachers no matter what. When I lived in Massachusetts, one studio paid me per student, with no base, and where class sizes were four to seven students per class, I regularly made twenty to thirty-five dollars per class. In some studios, depending on the state, yoga teachers are employees, but usually teachers are independent contractors, receiving no benefits including unemployment if a studio closes. Adri Frick, a studio owner in the Bay Area, said of this practice that "it saves the employers because they get to evade taxation law, and so they don't have to pay for workers comp. They also just save in accounting and administrative overhead by not keeping track of a lot of the finances."[4]

To balance this poor income from drop-in classes, many teachers teach workshops, retreats, and trainings, which bring in a greater income. With workshops, many studios offer teachers 60 or 70 percent of the profit. However, for a workshop to be successful, a teacher has to be well established and the content of their teaching desirable. Sometimes that demand matches the teacher's skill set and interests, but sometimes it doesn't. As you might imagine, more students are often interested in the physical dimensions of a practice than the philosophical or ethical ones. Handstand and arm balance workshops tend to do much better than workshops on compassion or consensual assists.

Thus, your beloved teacher is almost certainly underpaid! A yoga teaching career often only brings in $30,000 in annual income.[5] Teaching yoga is part of the gig economy, which 40 percent of workers are a part of.[6] Most studios don't take experience into account, so teachers with over a decade of experience are paid the same rate as those newly entering the field, unless they are a nationally famous teacher who can demand and receive a different arrangement.

I wonder: what is the impact over time of the teachers of the practice you love being devalued?

There are no data on how yoga teachers' incomes vary by gender, race, disability, and sexual orientation. But we do know, for the purposes of this book, that gay and bisexual men, who are often the most privileged members of the LGBTQ community, make 10 to 32 percent less than their straight counterparts. The average income for same-sex couples raising families is

$15,200, 20 percent less than other couples. Thirty-two percent of Black male same-sex couples and 28 percent of all female same-sex couples live below the poverty line.[7] I would imagine that the same (or worse) trends are found among yoga teachers who are queer, trans, people of color, disabled, and/or fat. And this affects our students as well, which I explore in the next section, since a twenty-dollar yoga class or two-thousand-dollar yoga retreat simply isn't accessible to many members of our community.

To be considered "successful" in yoga—to receive respect, to be invited to speak and teach at conferences, to bring your training to a given retreat center—a teacher must be profitable. What is considered "profitable" is intertwined with racism, transphobia, homophobia, fatphobia, and ableism, which includes the exoticization and tokenism of people of color, queer and trans folks, and working-class and disabled people, as well as their cultures. Despite many Black yoga teachers being students and teachers of yoga for decades, they are rarely asked to teach at prominent retreat centers or conferences. Despite yoga originating from South Asia, few conferences or trainings involve *any* South Asian teachers! Only one, if any, disabled person ever teaches at prominent conferences. Many retreat centers and magazine ads for trainings feature people of color, but does that truly represent who attends and teaches at those centers? Absolutely not!

Being a yoga teacher is a tough gig. You have to hustle. I have continued to teach because I deeply know the transformative potential of the teachings and see it as filling a gap in social justice work. For the majority of my career, I have had the privilege to continue teaching because I didn't have a child, student loans to pay off, or medical debt, and could make do on twelve classes per week that paid thirty to fifty dollars each, while subsidizing my income with retreats, trainings, and workshops. Many people I have trained with don't teach anymore or never taught full-time, because it couldn't sustain them financially. Thus, there are many people who have paid for and attended teacher trainings, are qualified to teach, and don't teach. Then why are we training so many to become teachers? So that those teaching the training can survive as yoga teachers.

Of course, teachers can teach outside of studio settings, renting space and doing marketing. Sometimes this is worthwhile and sustainable and welcomes people into the practice who wouldn't go to a gym or studio, and sometimes all the administration of teaching solo doesn't pay off in student attendance and therefore the financial well-being of the class. The benefit of teaching outside of a studio or gym is that a teacher and their students determine the culture of the space, such as valuing all bodies, offering a sliding-scale payment system, and focusing the practice on the physical, spiritual, or both. I have taught in countless spaces this way, in art galleries, nonprofit offices, event spaces, queer bars, and more. What is limited about this is that it can be difficult to attain new students. One of the advantages of teaching in a studio or gym, alongside other teachers, is that students take a class because it's at the right time or because they heard another student talk about a certain teacher being wonderful—this builds and builds until there is a lot of crossover between teachers and more of a community of practice.

Yoga Teacher Trainings

Yoga teacher trainings often cost between $4,000 and $12,000, and some occur over the course of one month. Furthermore, two hundred hours of training, $5,000, and a few months to learn the five-thousand-year-old practice of yoga is very little given the role that yoga teachers can play: philosopher, therapist, DJ, poet, choreographer, physical therapist, spiritual guide, visionary leader, and more. Each of these roles involves dedicated study, mentorship, and experience to execute well!

For many studios and retreat centers, yoga teacher trainings are the most lucrative aspect of their business. That in itself is not a problem. But we need to look at the motive in making money off of teacher trainings—is it to support other programming that is not as lucrative or to pay the rent? Or does the motive contain one of greed, counter to the practice of Asteya? A studio in East LA called The People's Yoga provides a yoga teacher training for $500, creating greater access and therefore a wider swath of potential teachers to draw from, with varied life experiences.

Historically, there has been no single path to teaching in yoga in India. There have been renunciates (*sanyasins*) who became teachers when their teacher recognized them as ready. Or a teacher would ask a student to teach because the teacher was approaching the end of their life or wanted to spread their teachings. Saints and sages sometimes are dedicated students who may be followed and requested to be teachers, without necessarily training or intending to teach. There are gurus, enlightened beings with experiential knowledge who may or may not have formal or academic training. *Acharyas* are teachers who studied the Vedas (ancient scriptures written in early Sanskrit revealed to seers and preserved through oral tradition) or in modern times have academic knowledge rather than experiential knowledge. The Brahman caste held householder and priestly duties, playing a role in rituals.

All of these paths to sharing yoga are vastly different from the fast-track two-hundred-hour model, which can take place over a time frame as short as one month or as long as a year. A student who graduates from a two-hundred-hour training doesn't necessarily continue as a mentee with their teachers and really doesn't have much accountability to anyone at all regarding what, how, and to whom they are teaching. This lack of accountability means that someone may make mistakes for which there is no recourse, unless the mistakes are egregious enough that they lose accreditation within Yoga Alliance or their lineage. This is very rare, though, as lineages tend to be insular and self-protecting, as explored in Matthew Remski's book *Practice and All Is Coming: Abuse, Cult Dynamics, and Healing in Yoga and Beyond.*

Tasha Eichenseher explained in a 2016 article in *Yoga Journal* that a search of marketing material from two-hundred-hour Yoga Alliance-registered yoga teacher trainings "turned up promises like graduates will learn pose modifications that are 'safe and effective for everybody,' will learn how to 'heal ourselves, our students, and the culture at large,' and will be able to 'register with Yoga Alliance and teach anywhere in the world,' with 'no further training required.' Broad declarations like these, along with the recent proliferation of [yoga teacher training] programs, have fueled a growing concern among teachers with decades of experience that yoga is losing its integrity."[8] The skills promised in these claims take a teacher a lifetime of personal practice and teaching practice to provide, not just a few months of study and a certificate.

As of 2016, there were 5,500 Yoga Alliance–registered yoga schools and 60,000 Yoga Alliance–registered teachers, which does not count some yoga schools that choose not to be affiliated with Yoga Alliance or that have their own training path toward teaching, such as Bikram or Iyengar. That is a lot of yoga teachers, and each school works with at least twenty students annually, producing hundreds of thousands of certified teachers with minimal training. Yoga is being practiced within offices and gyms and recommended by doctors and therapists, and there is great demand for yoga teachers and an assumption that we are all deeply trained and can easily adapt our skill set to the human in front of us. Doctors and therapists may recommend yoga without an understanding that there is a great variety of training and experience out there—not all teachers are skillful or have the necessary training for addressing a doctor's concerns.

At the same time, teacher training programs don't adequately prepare a teacher to skillfully teach the student with a shoulder separation, a replaced hip, a history of trauma, a fat, trans, or disabled body, or the depths of a practice like compassion. Timothy McCall, author of *Yoga as Medicine,* admits that there is a physical toll, a lack of well-trained teachers, and students trying to please teachers or "go hard" rather than be gentle and loving with their bodies. "They love their teachers and are gritting their teeth, saying they're fine, but then quietly going to the orthopedic surgeon. A teacher can encourage students not to do things they shouldn't be doing, but a lot of people will just do what they want."[9]

Our students trust us, and often they shouldn't. Many people have been injured in yoga classes, myself included, by teachers doing what they were trained to do or making an adjustment on someone that is not suitable and is actually harmful for the student. Teacher trainings rarely contain training on working with trauma, even though trauma is statistically bound to show up in yoga classrooms. Many yoga teachers teach outside of yoga studio or gym settings but often have no training themselves on working with the particular community they are teaching in, which a social worker in the same setting would be required to have.

The two-hundred-hour training model is not only not enough but really egregious, setting teachers up to fail, create harm, or both. Hopefully, someone who really wants to teach or work more deeply with a specific population gets trained, but they don't have to. There are three-hundred- and five-hundred- and now one-thousand-hour advanced yoga teacher training programs, and countless trainings on working with specific people: elders, incarcerated people, housing-insecure people, people with cancer, disabled people, folks with traumatic brain injuries, children, and so forth. I have taken many of these trainings, hungry for more knowledge and skills to meet my students with and in recognition that within the basic two hundred hours of training there isn't time to cover the vast applications of the practice for different populations and communities.

On the other side of the teacher training formula is the fact that many full-time yoga teachers who have been teaching for over a decade depend on the income of leading teacher trainings to sustain the rest of their offerings. In a workshop I attended with Andrew Tanner, co-author of *So You Want to Open a Yoga Studio,* he described daily classes as not income but marketing, and drew a pyramid that described workshops, retreats, and then teacher trainings bringing in greater and greater income. In offering yoga teacher trainings, there is an incentive to train anyone, to have a registration rather than an application for a training and to offer trainings as often as possible, which means pumping out yoga teachers with minimal skills who then compete against one another for jobs.

New yoga teachers sustain the industry of yoga, and some people pursue two-hundred-hour trainings because the teachings are intriguing and students often want more information. There are no easy answers, for we live in a capitalist society. But what if the goal were not profit, but integrity?

Yoga Stardom and the Cost of Yoga

Celebrity yoga teachers have made millions of dollars off of their teaching and cater to the upper class. Bikram Choudhury, founder of Bikram Yoga, earns $10 million per year.[10] John Friend, before he was brought down by his sexual misconduct with students, boasted 600,000 Anusara students.[11] Rodney Yee and Colleen Saidman Yee regularly host yoga retreats that cost more than $4,000 per student, not including airfare.[12] Former New York City studio Jivamukti Yoga ran yoga trainings that were a month long, with a 7:00 a.m. to 10:00 p.m. schedule, charging trainees $12,000.[13] Jois Yoga, a studio in Encinitas, cost over $1 million to build.[14] This catering to the owning class impacts the image and popular perception of yoga, for it is the owning class that controls marketing, can open boutique yoga studios that create the model of what a yoga studio is expected to be, and can attend yoga retreats around the world.

I am not at all opposed to wealthy, owning-class people attending yoga classes or retreats. I not only want them to but I think it is essential in order for our world to transform for those with the most power to really look at themselves and how they're living, and adjust accordingly, guided by the teachings of yoga. What is upsetting, and what I work against, is *catering* how yoga is offered in the US to those with class privilege, as it creates barriers for the rest of us and keeps yoga inaccessible to most people.

Yoga classes often cost between fifteen and twenty-five dollars for a sixty- to ninety-minute class. For some people this is a significant cost, especially if a student primarily practices or seeks to practice in a classroom setting. Many people have a strong home practice, not necessarily out of choice but because otherwise they could not practice yoga and they find such benefit to persevere on their own in this way. Though it is often said offhandedly that "yoga is for everyone," it is not yet playing out that way. Many of us are breaking the mold and finding creative ways to get yoga out to our own communities, but those efforts don't necessarily sustain teachers financially.

There are yoga teacher millionaires and underpaid teachers, some students can't pay to get in the door and other students have the capacity to pay for everyone to be there, some people feel entitled to practice and some teachers have to spend the first fifteen minutes of class explaining to their students why yoga is for them too. Part of the problem here is how we teach yoga, or what we do and do not teach as part of yoga. If we thoroughly taught and practiced the Yamas and Niyamas, the ethical practices and daily observances, we wouldn't have this vast discrepancy.

It's a well-proven fact that trickle-down economics doesn't work; the wealthy get wealthier and the poor get poorer. Trickle-down yoga doesn't work either. We have to change the whole structure so that everybody can practice yoga and the most marginalized are centered, knowing that when we do, freedom is available to everyone.

Retreats for the Wealthy

Everyone deserves peace of mind, everyone deserves a retreat, and everyone has had pain in their lives. Before teaching international yoga retreats, I thought of myself as committed to working with those who did not feel comfortable in a typical yoga classroom, and I thought I would never want to work intensively with those who feel comfortable and welcome every time they enter a yoga studio. What I realize now is that part of my judgment, prejudice, and comparison was my own trauma around classism. As a result of growing up working class and being harmed personally by wealthy people, I had created separation between those with wealth and myself. I had never wanted to work with those with wealth; rather, I wanted to work with those who face daily oppression and struggle. I had dehumanized the wealthy. And as the path of yoga takes us on, in teaching these retreats, I chose to heal.

Many teachers offer retreats as a way to be paid to teach somewhere beautiful and to make money in a short time. Although I never made this much, it's fairly common for teachers to make $20,000 in a one-week retreat.[15] Given that the average annual salary for yoga teachers is $37,000, this goes a long way and can allow teaching yoga to be sustainable. However, yoga teachers need to check this by our practice—how much is enough? When does a skillful business acumen wander into greed? What corners might we be cutting in an effort to make profit? What is the intention?

When I taught my first retreat in Tulum, Mexico, I received an email from a friend and colleague. She claimed that I was selling out, teaching yoga on the beach yet neglecting the injustice done to the Mayan community in Tulum, providing "fantasy travel" to white upper-class US citizens. She thought that I was creating more harm than good, writing of her commitment to racial justice and her disappointment in my retreat being purely about yoga without an underlying justice motive. This was an opportunity to practice self-reflection, or *svadhyaya,* one of the Niyamas of the eight limbs of Raja Yoga.

I try to offer my retreats at host sites owned by the people of that country—a worker-owned cooperative retreat center would be my dream. I teach about lovingkindness, compassion, forgiveness, joy, and equanimity, which lead to both individual and collective liberation. In my dharma talks on these topics, I quote revolutionary leaders, artists, and thinkers. I am teaching the dharma of transformation, which I believe will lead to a kinder, more honest world. I offer payment options and set my prices low, and I always teach with a co-teacher who has a different identity.

I do not offer a service component to my yoga retreats because there have been many studies that demonstrate that doing service for a community for a few hours a day for a week, known as "voluntourism," creates more harm than good: volunteers fill local jobs, taking the place of local people who would be paid a salary; the skills of volunteers don't necessarily match the needs of the local community; there is no long-term commitment to sustain the offering made by volunteering; and it can perpetuate the "white savior complex," the idea that white people are essential to Black and Brown people's survival.[16] Instead, I donate 10 percent of my earnings to local justice work wherever I work.

In the annual retreats that I have taught in beautiful places in other countries, I have worked with people positioned like those who have harmed me, and in the process I have healed my own trauma around class. I have learned to see my students who can afford these retreats as human beings struggling with patience, discipline, relationships, self-care, and connection, just like me. I also have come to understand the wisdom of the Buddhist adage that "hurt people hurt people." If we mix power into this equation, it can become a devastating formula, for a hurting wealthy person can wreak havoc and destroy lives en masse through policy, trade agreements, the training of police officers, the construction of weapons, or the polluting of a water supply, in ways that people without power simply cannot. Thus, in bringing these transformational practices of compassion, forgiveness, and lovingkindness to those with power, the potential to intervene in mass harm is great.

I bring my whole self into these retreats; I am honest about who I am and the struggles in my life and how the dharma has taught me how to live in a way that creates the least harm possible. This becomes an asset to the retreats, for my students get to learn the teachings from a unique perspective that they likely haven't been exposed to in their lives. I do not put

myself in such a position often, for I have learned that doing so is depleting, but once a year is manageable to take on this role. I have learned how
to skillfully unveil my trans identity in my dharma talks and how to set
boundaries when questions become too personal or invasive.

The price that I set for these international retreats is quite low compared to common rates for yoga retreats—weeklong retreats often sell for
$2,000 to $4,000. I wasn't trying to make the most money possible—I was
trying to get away from New York, be somewhere beautiful, and immerse
my students in the practice. As a result, teachers, restaurant managers, post
office clerks, nonprofit workers, burlesque dancers, and nurses who often
can't afford a retreat attended my retreats alongside the owners of poetry
journals and art galleries, managers for famous musicians, and successful
New York real estate agents.

Everyone can benefit from the teachings. The problem is not that
wealthy people can go on retreat, self-reflect, and return more grounded
and purposeful. It's that everyone else can't necessarily do it. Not all retreats
are transformative—some focus exclusively on the physical practice—but
we exercise faith in the teachings and offer them up to those with power.
The work is to provide access to yoga in a myriad of ways, not to cease
retreats that center around transformative teachings.

⁓

In 2020, as the pandemic bore down on us, it left many yoga teachers out of work, no longer able to teach in person. As Yoga Alliance had
meetings and consultations on how to support teachers, an organization
called Reclamation Ventures rose up. They offered an initial grant of "unre-
stricted funding" to 101 wellness practitioners, with over 2,700 applicants,
prioritizing practitioners who were people of color, queer, and/or disabled.
In their first round, they gave a total of $169,080, with another round set to
be distributed in August. Recipients would use the grants for immediate
relief, such as for rent or groceries. Of the recipients, 73 percent were people
of color, 36 percent were LGBTQ, 8 percent were impacted by the criminal
justice system, and 8 percent were immigrants.[17] Reclamation Ventures was
ready to act, formed the previous year to support wellness practitioners

from targeted populations in making their offerings accessible. This is what yoga could do—action born out of our individual and collective practice of love and integrity, using the money in the wellness industry to support those most vulnerable in thriving and the communities they come from in accessing wellness services.

Yoga is a practice and a large industry. What does yoga sell? The market of yoga can reinforce oppression in our world, or it can be a tool to interrupt, redirect, and reallocate. The Yamas and Niyamas, if practiced with depth and breadth, can be anti-capitalist in nature. Therefore, in the pursuit of justice, practicing and teaching the Yamas and Niyamas is important not just for individuals but also for the potential impact. Individuals, studios, yoga clothing companies, yoga mat companies, yoga service organizations, and teacher training programs make choices that can align with capitalism or align with yoga. For yoga teachers, part of our practice is to earn what we are worth, while considering what is enough. For teachers with marginalized identities, it can be some deep work to demand and claim our worth; for teachers with privilege, it can be some deep work to let go of some of the market share and settle for "enough." May we use the energy of money for good, for the benefit of all, for justice, for liberation, for repair, and for redistribution, in daily small ways and in supporting great, profound action and policy.

CULTURAL APPROPRIATION
AND YOGA

I CANNOT WRITE about yoga without writing about cultural appropriation, out of my own practices of Ahimsa, Satya, and Asteya. Part of how I came to be practicing yoga and writing this book is due to how I benefited from the colonization of India, as well as modern global capitalist and globalization projects all over the world. Out of compassion for those who have been taken from for many generations, writing about this dynamic and my benefiting from it is the least I can do. Out of my own commitment to not add harm to a world already greatly hurting, I need to write about this pertinent topic. The process of engaging this topic is not easy; there is no clear "right" and "wrong," it's not about "getting it" or having answers. But engaging in the conversation about the role of cultural appropriation in yoga is essential to practicing truthfulness, determination, compassion, and forgiveness. The only way is through, and the more we resist this conversation the greater the suffering becomes.

Cultural appropriation is the taking of aspects of another culture and using them for profit or personal gain. Maisha Z. Johnson of Everyday Feminism says, "Cultural appropriation is a process that takes a traditional practice from a marginalized group and turns it into something that benefits the dominant group—ultimately erasing its origins and meaning."[1] Yoga in the

US, and arguably around the world, is financially benefitting people without an ancestral connection to yoga, and certainly financially benefitting white people most of all. Temple University professor Olufunmilayo Arewa says, "In some instances, a line is crossed and cultural borrowing can become exploitative. Crossing this line may turn acts of borrowing into cultural appropriation. Context, particularly as it relates to power relationships, is a key factor in distinguishing borrowing from exploitative cultural appropriation."[2]

Some yoga studios use Indian and Hindu cultural items and artifacts to signify authenticity and authority, without necessarily having a connection to those artifacts or an understanding of why they have them in their space or their logo. I have witnessed countless examples of this. A prominent studio in New York had a "bindi bar"; yoga clothing companies put Ganesha or the Om symbol on the butt of pants; white *kirtan* singers mispronounce Sanskrit. And the opposite is also true—some studios laud offering yoga with no Sanskrit, no chanting, and even no *pranayama*—just using yogic asanas devoid of any connection to the history and roots of yoga. Susanna Barkataki offers, "If someone from the dominant culture completes a yoga teacher training that is primarily asana based, and remains blissfully unaware of the complexity of yoga's true aim or the roots of the practice, they are culturally appropriating yoga. By remaining unaware of the history, roots, complexity, and challenges of the heritage from which yoga springs and the challenges it has faced under Western culture, they perpetuate a re-colonization of it by stripping its essence away."[3]

I do not know all there is to know about the colonization of India or all of the ways that yoga and Buddhism were taken from (or offered by) South Asian peoples. I understand that the story is complex. Some South Asian teachers offered the teachings up to people in Britain, the US, and other imperialist countries, out of a concern that the teachings would otherwise be lost to the world, so grave and threatening to the continued existence of the practice were the conditions of colonization. This offering from South Asian teachers was an act of resistance to the violence on their continent. White people also went to India and brought the practices back to their home countries, sometimes humbly so at the suggestion of their teachers and sometimes with ego and ambition. Sheena Sood warns,

"Yogis—especially those who hope to offer yoga as a tool for fueling resilience and resistance in our movements—must be critical of the trendy popularization of yoga. Yoga circulates as a global commodity through white supremacy, neoliberalism and capitalism."[4] Tracing back how convert yogis encountered the practices is important and complicated, yet is rarely offered by yoga teacher trainings. It is important that convert yoga teachers consider (over and over again through years of teaching) their intention in offering up yoga, commit to studentship and resist labels of expertise, and delve into racial justice and accountability practices.

Susanna Barkataki opens an article entitled "How to Decolonize Your Yoga Practice" with this reflection: "As an Indian woman living in the U.S. I've often felt uncomfortable in many yoga spaces. At times, such as when I take a $25.00 yoga class by a well-known teacher who wants to 'expose us to the culture by chanting Om to start class' and her studio hangs the Om symbol in the wrong direction, my culture is being stripped of its meaning and sold back to me in forms that feel humiliating at best and dehumanizing at worst."[5] This is the impact of cultural appropriation, in a daily way, on many people of the Indian diaspora, and out of compassion and an understanding of interdependence I suggest that the rest of us stop and listen.

For many convert yogis, yogis without an ancestral connection to the practice, the phrase *cultural appropriation* can create resistance, denial, and avoidance—because it sheds light on the violence and ensuing suffering over a hundred years of the process of Britain "conquering" and colonizing India. Cultural appropriation is taking a ritual or traditional practice out of its original geographic site and context and resurfacing it elsewhere, often devoid of its original significance and intention. Those who take the practice benefit culturally and often financially. Those who experience their own cultural practice being taken are rarely given intellectual, cultural, or financial recognition, and are even pathologized or surveilled due to these practices, or fetishized and put on a pedestal.[6] In the process of British colonization, practitioners of yoga and Ayurveda in India were maimed, killed, and demonized and sacred, ancient texts were burned, as a way to erode the spirit of the Indian people in the interest of making them easier to conquer, colonize, and govern. Indeed, this practice is powerful, and as seen in other processes of colonization around the world, taking, vilifying, and destroying languages and spiritual and cultural practices takes generations to heal and repair.

Many yoga teachers coming out of yoga teacher trainings are familiar with breaths and postures but do not know the history of how they came to study yoga or their own lineage of learning the teachings beyond the teacher they learned from directly, nor are they familiar with the great teachers from India or even that it is a six-thousand-year-old practice. Yoga in the US and Canada is primarily Raja Yoga and prioritizes the postural practice and neglects the other seven limbs, such that people unfamiliar with yoga associate it with exercise. This is particularly alarming and upsetting within the context of yoga because the teachings of yoga cultivate nonviolence, integrity, honesty, nonattachment, and union, and the breath and meditative practices impact the nervous system and emotional intelligence. The cultural appropriation of yoga is a practice of greed, separation, violence, alienation, and dehumanization—very much unyogic! Sheena Sood shares, "Hindus and Western yogis perpetuate the violence of yoga through bypassing the moral tenets for a disembodied, posture-heavy practice that presents a surface-level understanding of humanity's interconnectedness in suffering and liberation."[7]

Generations of South Asian people living in the US and all over the world who want to access the teachings of their own cultural heritage cannot afford it or do not feel comfortable in the spaces where it is offered due to incessant microaggressions and institutional racism, among other oppressive dynamics often present in yoga spaces. South Asian folks encounter these dynamics as both practitioners and teachers and are often heartbroken and outraged by their culture being misunderstood, misrepresented, tokenized, and dismissed. That the yoga industry purports to be about healing yet is averse to evolving and transforming as an industry when called out or called in, continuing to perpetuate the same harm, exacerbates the wound felt by South Asian folks. Most South Asian people, just like most trans, disabled, Black, and/or fat people, have stories of this exclusion and harm within yoga. Sheena Sood describes her experience, writing, "I often left feeling awkward and angered about how unwelcome I felt practicing in such culturally appropriated yogic settings."[8] Very rarely are South Asian yogis lifted up as great teachers currently within yoga in the US, and when they are, they are often tokenized—lifted up without the conference or retreat center doing real groundwork to contextualize and create relationships for and with that teacher so that it feels good and is beneficial to both teachers and students to share and learn from the teachings. When a South Asian teacher challenges a white teacher's racism, they are most often met with defensiveness, surprise at being called out, blame, shame, and white fragility while enduring harassment and risking job security. Lakshmi Nair shares, "Working as an Indian-American yoga teacher has been deeply challenging on so many levels. Yoga has been a spiritual anchor for me, a root that tethers me to this Earth from a specific cultural location. To find that often there is no place for me in what is supposed to be the spiritual tradition of my ancestors has often left me feeling adrift."[9]

It can be difficult for white yogis or those without a cultural and ethnic connection to yoga to come to terms with cultural appropriation and the anger and grief of those harmed by it, because so many of us practitioners and teachers have been transformed by yogic teachings and intend no harm. We may become afraid that we are being asked to give up our participation in these practices, or that our participation at all is wrong. We may feel under attack and therefore hold even tighter to these practices, engage in immense resistance to those speaking about cultural appropriation, or cease the practice altogether, unwilling to reside in a complicated relationship with the teachings and their political context in South Asia.

As recognized in so many social justice workshops, intent is different than impact, and it's important to both hold the goodness of one's intent while being accountable for any harmful impact, regardless of the intent. If, as yoga practitioners, we are committed to nonviolence and integrity, the first two practices of the first limb of yoga, then out of our commitment to the teachings that we cherish we must examine this, look at ourselves, and consider the route by which the practices arrived in our lives. We must examine who is uplifted as the great yoga teachers of our day and how that recognition intersects with the exclusion of South Asian teachers, cultural appropriation, the tokenism of recognizing one South Asian teacher here or there, or the exoticization of South Asian teachers that presumes their wisdom based on their identity rather than their practice. As teachers and practitioners of yoga or meditation, we must study the current and historical politics of India and the impact of British colonization on the various strata of Indian society and on the yogic teachings in particular. Susanna Barkataki offers, "Yoga means liberation from every construct, including that of race, gender, time, space, location, identity, and even history itself. However, in the current cultural context where there is a billion-dollar industry profiting off taking yoga out of context, branding and repackaging it for monetary gain, we need to address this. Or else we perpetuate a second colonization, i.e., eventually eradicating the true practice, as was accomplished in many places under Britain's occupation of India, and we stray further on the path of maya, or illusion."[10]

Some white yoga teachers have learned about cultural appropriation and ceased teaching. This is one route to take, but for me it doesn't sit well. It feels like abdicating personal responsibility while the larger institutional harm continues. I know that if I were to stop teaching, the cultural appropriation of yoga would continue. If white anti-racist yogis were to stop teaching, the white folks who feel no accountability and are perfectly content profiting and gaining cultural capital from the practice would continue doing just that.

I am in a better position to interrupt and educate my fellow white yogis while I continue to teach, and to teach in a way that models some interruptions. And I love the practice: it has provided the precise tools that I needed countless times, and I see it making practitioners better people. Thus, my route is to continue to humbly practice and teach in an anti-racist way, invite and receive feedback, and maintain relationships with South Asian colleagues as well as fellow anti-racist white folks.

The Hindu Right, Casteism, and Yoga

An important consideration within the realm of cultural appropriation is the way in which yoga has been taken up by the Hindu Right in India as a tool to further oppress Muslims, Dalits, Adivasi people, queer folks, and Christians, claiming yoga to specifically have Hindu roots, which is false and misleading. Before British colonization, India was not a monolithic country, and many religions and spiritual practices existed on the subcontinent, sometimes peacefully, sometimes not; there were many overlapping strands of Indigenous practices that were consolidated into Hinduism by British colonizers; there was no India and no Pakistan. The 1947 partition occurring on the eve of independence from Britain displaced many Muslims into Pakistan and many Sikhs and Hindus into present-day India. Since the start of these nation-states, their relationship has been marked by contempt, conflict, cultural dissonance, and war. Claiming sole ownership of spiritual practices (such as yoga, Ayurveda, and Unani medicine) that were once shared and overlapped among different cultural and religious groups living in the same land is a product of colonization and partition. The Hindu Right is currently claiming the practice of yoga as a specifically Hindu practice. Some yoga festivals put on by the Hindu Right in India have been held on sacred sites of desecrated Muslim temples. "International Yoga Day" on June 21 was brought to the United Nations by Narendra Modi as prime minister of India and member of the Bharatiya Janata Party, a right-wing Hindu nationalist party.

On US soil, the Hindu American Foundation (HAF) has a "Take Back Yoga" campaign that insists that yoga is authentically Hindu. HAF warns against anti-Hindu hate crimes in India, while Muslims actually face the greatest threat for their religious practices. Through the Take Yoga Back campaign, HAF gains legitimacy that they use toward supporting the Islamophobic Hindu Right. Prachi Patankar warns, "Claiming that yoga belongs to Hinduism—or even to India or South Asia, for that matter—assumes the origins and evolution of yoga as monolithic. Neither contemporary 'yoga' nor 'Hinduism' is age-old or homogenous. Actually, both were assembled in the nineteenth and twentieth centuries, in interaction with British colonial realities.... Caste-privileged Hindu leaders, through violent domination, have culturally appropriated a variety of diverse sects, practices, beliefs, and rituals that have existed for centuries."[11]

Yoga practitioners must also grapple with the legacy of casteism, which shows up within yoga as well. Casteism is present within some often-used texts such as the Yoga Sutras, as well as the Sanskrit language itself being reserved for the Brahman caste, which is something for any yoga practitioner to grapple with. My colleague nisha ahuja acknowledges that "casteism has led to violence and the exclusion of people being denied access to spiritual teachings and spaces, while also denying the spiritual practices, rituals, and traditions that come from Dalit and Adivasi peoples. Their practices have been historically co-opted into mainstream Hindu practices, including some yogic practices and philosophies."[12] Prachi Patankar writes in her article reflecting on South Asian reactions to cultural appropriation, "As someone from a Bahujan (lower-caste) farmer family in rural India, 'yoga' was something very distant to me. It lived in the culture of the brahmanic upper middle class of urban India. Only recently, I have seen formal yoga being introduced into the vocabulary of the people I grew up with, and see 'yoga mats' for sale in stores in some of the bigger towns near my village."[13] The practices offered by yoga are not politically neutral, and don't necessarily inevitably lead toward liberation. Like any tool, the potent practices can be used for harm or healing.

From an upper-caste Hindu-Punjabi family, Sheena Sood shares about her inheritance of the positions of both oppressor and victim: "I have sought guidance in decolonizing my ancestors' spiritual traditions. However, this journey has not been a one-way voyage of merely seeing my ancestors as perpetual victims of colonial misappropriation. It has also meant seeing my ancestors as perpetrators of oppressive harm and awakening to the realization that in order for these healing traditions to be purposed toward embodied freedom for all of humanity and Mother Earth, they must be wholly decolonized from the interlocking logics of settler colonialism, racialized slavery and Orientalism (Smith 2012), as well as from the structures that uphold Hindutva and Brahmanical supremacist ideologies."

Not being taught the modern political context of yoga within India or the political history preceding, including, and following colonization, many students and teachers simply don't know about the ways in which casteism is present in yoga or the political claims to yoga. Hundreds of us celebrate International Yoga Day in Times Square and imagine that it is politically neutral. My friend Ashwin Manthripragada reflects, "When my white friends who are yoga teachers ask me about cultural appropriation, I'm just like, there's no monolithic culture to appropriate from. And yoga itself just means connection. There are many kinds and it has been evolving over a long time. And yes, Sanskrit, Brahmanical thought and knowledge, and power and privilege are all implicated."[14] Cultural appropriation, casteism, and battles over who owns yoga are part of our inheritance as yogis. How can we continue to recognize and heal the harm within our lineages and bend the practice toward justice?

Important Practices in Countering Cultural Appropriation

Addressing cultural appropriation within our yoga practice takes effort. What follows is by no means exhaustive; rather, it's a set of ever-evolving practices that keep me accountable to embodying the liberatory potential of yoga. I have learned and taken on many of the below practices through workshops and articles generously offered by South Asian colleagues, scholars, and yoga teachers such as nisha ahuja, Susanna Barkataki, Andrea Jain, Sheena Sood, Tejal Patel, Jesal Parikh, Anurag Gupta, and Lakshmi Nair, all of whom extend requests and invitations to be more equitable and accountable to those with an ancestral connection to yoga. Rarely do yoga teacher trainings contain these discussions, so graduates of those trainings continue to perpetuate and even expand their cultural appropriation. I believe in the basic goodness of each teacher and practitioner, and it is from that place that I offer up these practices that have resonated for me and have allowed me to earn the trust and respect of South Asian colleagues.

In work that seeks to counter cultural appropriation, often the term *decolonizing* is used. It's important to deeply consider what we mean, and what actions are required. Wayne Yang and Eve Tuck, in their article "Decolonizing Is Not a Metaphor," offer up that what is wanted is what was taken— land, spiritual and cultural practices, language. They argue, "Decolonization brings about the repatriation of Indigenous land and life."[15] Decolonization is unsettling, and it does not happen unnoticed. Hopefully, then, some of these practices are unsettling to the industry of yoga, and offer up benefits, livelihood, and opportunities to South Asian people.

Before her own list of best practices, Sheena Sood offers these instructions in absorbing her suggestions: "Consider reading these principles in the most embodied way available to you—perhaps slowly at your altar, in a sacred space, with a group of close comrades, or in a yoga class. If you can, pause in between reading each principle, and take a deep breath on the interims. Allow yourself to notice where you feel each word and syllable landing, where discomfort arises, and where freedom expands as you peruse the list. These sacred breaths are the first intentions toward embodying a decolonized yoga."[16]

These practices may be useful for convert yogis and those with an ancestral connection to yoga, for again, yogic practices are a tool that can be used to perpetrate harm (such as soldiers being taught meditation and yogic breathing to become more astute shooters) or create healing. This list will be ever evolving, as the practice is, as humanity is. We will never be complete with liberation, but what a lofty goal, inwardly and outwardly! Please try them on, share and discuss them, and improve upon them.

Humility

I have learned from many South Asian colleagues a profound humility, for many of them consider themselves but one drop of wisdom in the ocean of wisdom and profess their own continuing studentship. It is indeed a wise practice to resist calling anyone an "expert" or even a "teacher," including ourselves, and continuously honor our studentship. It's been said that you can't "teach yoga"—that yoga is a process for each individual and community, one of unifying and intimacy. This humility counters the pedestal many yoga teachers are placed on or willingly occupy, and I believe it is better for both students and the teacher in the long run. In my years of teaching yoga and witnessing many teachers' sexual violence tear apart the community, I know that their willing occupation of the teacher pedestal and lack of horizontal accountability contribute to the problem. When we practice humility even in the offering of yoga, refusing to be the authority but rather directing students to their own inner authority, we honor the practice and the expertise of the student, and we expose the gaps in a teacher's own knowledge and practice.

Generosity and Gratitude

As previously discussed in the chapter on joy, generosity was the first practice given to lay practitioners by the Buddha, and it is enormously important in social justice, countering the capitalist impulse to take, take, take, and more, more, more. My gratitude for the practice is expressed through my words, my financial decisions, and my relationships. Generosity and gratitude are practices by which I acknowledge and thank those from whom I learned the teachings, as well as the places and teachers from whom the teachings originally came, and commit to passing on the teachings with integrity.

I work to have sangha, or spiritual community, with an array of people who can affirm, inspire, and challenge my practice. These colleagues and friends generously hold me accountable when I run astray of the teachings or practices; such relationships allow me to grow and evolve. Drawing from social justice group agreements of "move up, move back," I work to recognize the space that I take up as a white person who is often assumed to be a man and how that may impact others in the space, and move back as a practice of generosity.

I work to be welcoming and extend extra effort to those who may feel uncomfortable in a yoga classroom or training, to really invite them in and co-create their belonging. I also recognize that I may trigger someone in different ways—not because of who I am in my heart but because of my physical form and my positionality in greater systems of power and domination. In the moment of my identity, positionality, and embodiment triggering someone, my practice is to validate their experience, to remain soft and open, and to listen.

Yoga Is Not Just Physical

I say this to my students every time I teach. Patty Adams, a white queer yoga teacher in Durham, North Carolina, says, "I teach on themes, always exploring physical postures that mirror spiritual postures."[17] Yoga asana is a small component of the larger practice, and it is also a doorway for many people to the deeper teachings. When we talk about yoga and we're talking about the physical practice, can we specifically name that as asana practice, and not yoga, as if the physical is the whole of the practice? Yoga as a whole, encompassing ethical practices, daily observances, breath practices, physical postures, and meditation, invites us into a deeper way of being.

What does it mean if someone asks, "Do you do yoga?" Are you a steward of love and truth in this world? Do you use your breath for self-regulation of your nervous system? Do you reflect on your words and actions daily to ensure that they align with the Yamas? We can each challenge the popular notion of asanas encompassing the whole of yoga, which strips incredible richness from the practice.

Learning and Respecting Cultural Practices

We can cite cultural references as we attempt to understand and connect with the complexity, culture, and history that birthed yoga. If you use sacred objects, such as an Om symbol or a statue of the Hindu goddess Lakshmi, treat them with respect as defined by the culture they come from, and know their meaning, significance, and story. Hanging the Om symbol upside down, displaying Om on the butt of yoga pants, decorating a toilet with a statue of the Hindu god Hanuman, or having the Hindu goddess Saraswati on your altar but knowing nothing about her are forms of cultural appropriation. Practice cultural appreciation, study up, and only move forward when you're sure of the integrity of your action.

When using Sanskrit, learn how to pronounce it, and know what you are saying and why you're using it. When nisha ahuja is leading a yoga session using Sanskrit, she lets people know that they will be using it and what the meanings of the words are, while also contextualizing the caste and religious divides that Sanskrit arises out of. She offers the intention of using Sanskrit to engage the energy channels of the physical and subtle bodies.

Reparations

As a white person practicing and teaching yoga, part of my Yamas practice is reparations. Yoga is not my cultural inheritance, and many of my ancestors were British. "Reparations campaigns encompass a wide array of demands. Most commonly, reparations in our contemporary movements are justified by the historical pains and damage caused by European settler colonialism and are proposed in the form of demands for financial restitution, land redistribution, political self-determination, culturally relevant education programs, language recuperation, and the right to return (or repatriation)," writes Black Lives Matter co-founder Patrisse Cullors.[18]

Susanna Barkataki writes that reparations involve "atoning for what has been stolen and returning many of the benefits, rights and profits of a culture's inheritance to its creators and culture."[19] A practice that my colleague Molly Kitchen and I utilized in the two years that we co-led a yoga teacher training was to invite our trainees and drop-in students to donate to a South Asian–led organization while also pledging a set amount to that organization ourselves, giving it a line in our training's budget. We recognized that we were two white people making a living teaching yoga and training others in how to teach yoga, and we wanted that very offering to benefit those with an ancestral connection to yoga. We made posters and handouts profiling the organizations we were donating to each month, and let our trainees know how much we collectively raised for each organization. Out of the practice of *dana,* or generosity, we considered an amount that we could dedicate each month that was a stretch—a little out of range, a little uncomfortable, as is customary in Buddhist retreats utilizing dana to support teachers.

Molly shares,

A donation cannot abolish our participation in cultural appropriation. A monetary offering was just one humble starting point. For me, it also meant researching about the South Asian community organizations we were donating to, learning what their struggles and celebrations were. And for the folks that attend our classes, it was an important conversation starter that encouraged further study about the history of yoga and the possibility of practicing in a socially and culturally responsible way. Rather than just being a cash gift, we did our best to have the donations be a conversation starter and learning opportunity for our largely white student body, so they could have resources for practicing in a more culturally-aware way.[20]

Convert yogis can also surrender opportunities to skilled teachers with an ancestral connection to yoga or refuse to teach in a training or conference where there aren't at least five South Asian teachers. In doing this, we leverage our privilege. This can extend to people of other marginalized and targeted backgrounds as well, such as disabled yogis, fat yogis, trans yogis, Black yogis, and more.

My hope is that the yoga industry can come to this practice as a whole and dedicate real financial resources to the people whose very ancestors created the practice of yoga, and that South Asian people can continue to benefit from yoga, whether they are involved in the yoga industry or not.

Difficult Questions

In so many yoga trainings, I am the annoying critical queer asking all the hard questions. I have been raised by social justice movements, and for better and worse I have cultivated critique! I am also partnered with a gender studies and disability studies scholar and professor, who counters my hard questions with even more challenging questions. Susanna Barkat-aki recommends asking and receiving hard questions in her list of practices to counter cultural appropriation.[21] These questions are necessary in the yoga world in order to truly practice liberatory yoga.

We need to ask who is most able to access yoga today and how that might be a legacy of past injustices. We need to assess how we can address those injustices in our lives and practice. Notice who is present in a yoga space and who is not, and what that communicates about who feels mirrored, safe, represented, and seen in that space. Notice who is not there, and through the depth of your truthfulness practice be honest about the ableism, racism, transphobia, or fatphobia that keeps people out of the room or training. And not all spaces are for everyone. Not many white teachers can skillfully hold the hearts and lineages of a room of people of color—so those of us who are white need to support other teachers who are skilled to hold that space while doing our own work on our participation in systems of oppression.

We also need to be open to critical feedback, seeing it as an opportunity to grow rather than an insult or critique on our person. If someone points out that you could do your yoga practice differently to avoid the harm of cultural appropriation, listen up! As nisha puts it, this is "an invitation to learn how to love bigger."

LIBERATORY MODELS OF
YOGA AND BUDDHISM

WHILE A CRITIQUE of the mainstream and status quo is important, it is equally or perhaps even more important to have liberatory models. I have begun to see critiques as noticing gaps that need to be filled—sometimes with passion and anger, other times with creativity and curiosity, and often both. There will always be gaps, and they will always need filling. It is the nature of our humanity to be imperfect, and so are the institutions that we create. It is not necessarily a failure; it is natural and inevitable. It is courageous work to create organizations, projects, and trainings that aspire to create a new model that makes the old model seem obsolete, while inviting feedback and committing to continued evolution. All projects will have gaps. We learn from the mistakes and what is missing, and we take the lesson to create something more complete, based on the moment that we are in, which will also be incomplete.

I co-founded Third Root Community Health Center because there were few social justice organizations at the time taking on healing and few holistic healing businesses centering social justice. Social justice organizations had no time for healing or restoration, and healing businesses had little patience or courage for conversations about dynamics of privilege and oppression as integral to the potential of healing. It was a gap, and between

Third Root co-founder Green Wayland-Llewellin and I, we had the healing practices, courage, vision, skills, and network to get something off the ground. Third Root was a collective project, and the co-owners, teachers, practitioners, clients, and community members over thirteen years of business shaped it, making it so much better than it was initially! Third Root always had gaps, and there are now many organizations focused on the nexus of social justice and healing that do what we set out to do better than we have done it. I bow deeply to those organizations, and I have learned from the many critiques of Third Root.

I find it important to be familiar with projects structured by the teachings of yoga and Buddhism and familiar with where that is written into how we show up and what we do—especially when things break down—and how we involve practitioners who are likewise committed to kindness, integrity, social justice, and growth. Larry Yang offers, "Beloved communities are envisioned as those that embody the values of love and justice in every aspect of their being, even when circumstances are difficult or oppressive. A Beloved Community assumes that all our lives are interrelated and the social nature of our humanity is not secondary to any other aspect of life."[1]

In this chapter, I discuss three impactful projects among hundreds to choose from, diving into the love and liberation they are driven by, how they create buy-in from the community they are working with, the effects or evidence of the practice on their students and sanghas, and the resistance and struggles that they have faced. I spoke to Andres Gonzalez of the Holistic Life Foundation in Baltimore, Nikki Myers of Yoga of 12-Step Recovery, and Brenda Salgado of East Bay Meditation Center about their work, while also researching the organizations and articles and news pieces created about each of them. I regard these leaders as my comrades and members of my sangha.

Yoga is often associated with just the postural practices and Buddhism is often regarded as a training for the mind. However, yoga is so much more than physical, and Buddhism includes the body as well as ethics, heart practices, and a road map for life. These projects embody that deeper expansive practice, using the tools for individual and community liberation. They consider the inner and outer worlds to be mirrors of each other, dependent upon one another; we can't have communities of love until we are filled with deep, radical love for all people in our bodies, minds, and hearts. And we can't be truly at peace in our heartminds when our communities are bombarded by state violence, neglect, and poverty.

The Holistic Life Foundation (HLF) offers yoga in Baltimore public schools and conducts presentations about yoga and mindfulness in schools as one of the longest-standing organizations in the field. Many of HLF's students have become teachers, and the three co-founders, Andres Gonzalez, Ali Smith, and Atman Smith, have begun leading from behind. In some schools, HLF has a yoga room, in other schools, HLF leaders show up to teach regular classes. I interviewed Andres Gonzalez.

Yoga of 12-Step Recovery (Y12SR) offers leadership trainings around the world, training local leaders in using yoga as a vital tool in addiction recovery. The organization holds an annual leaders' retreat, co-organizes a yoga and recovery conference on each US coast, and supports graduates in running their own weekly classes. I interviewed Nikki Myers, the founder of Y12SR.

The East Bay Meditation Center (EBMC) came into being by asking "what is missing" in contemporary Buddhism and trying to fill those gaps. They are located in downtown Oakland, California, and have uplifted some of the most well-known teachers who are LGBTQ and/or people of color over the years. They have the longest-enduring weekly sitting group for people of color, as well as an Alphabet Sangha for LGBTQ folks, an Every Body Every Mind sangha for people with disabilities, and programs for teens, people in recovery, and families. They are specifically oriented around social justice and uniquely require that every teaching team involve a person of color. I interviewed Brenda Salgado, a former executive director at EBMC.

Purpose and Practice

Each of these organizations are in practice, constantly and humbly improving. The practice lives through these three leaders, which becomes their purpose as individuals, and they have joined together with like-minded people committed to practice to form their organizations, which then becomes a collective practice.

Andres Gonzalez states the purpose of HLF in Baltimore schools as "reminding [our students] of the tools for resilience that they have for self-regulation and health, physically and mentally." Nikki Myers describes Yoga of 12-Step Recovery, founded in 2004, as looking "at all of yoga, the bigger definition of yoga, [bigger] than even 'tools,' beyond tools." She continues, "Yoga gives us a way to deepen at the level of energy, awareness. The 12-step program gives us a way to structurally and cognitively look at patterns. I assert that there may be a way to use the process in 12-step programs to address some of the bigger things—sooner or later we have to look at the bigger stuff. It's about deeper and deeper levels of awareness in order to create self- and collective transformation." Yoga philosophy is written into the purpose and practices of these organizations, and it guides them in their own growth and evolution. Brenda Salgado shared, "EBMC is a place where you can be around people who have experienced your particular suffering in the world, to discover a sense of wholeness and dignity that is present with you no matter where you are. Not necessarily a place to stay, but to heal."

For HLF, the yoga is in the relationship, the connection—meeting children and youth where they are at and equipping them with tools relevant for their lives. Andres says,

> We go in and frame [yoga] as a survival skill, ways to manage yourself, to take care of yourself. Youth we deal with have extreme heightened senses all the time. When you can show them how to take themselves to a calm place, they're like, wow, I want to go there instead, because my home life sucks. When you tell them, "I was in your shoes, this will help you in any endeavor, practical tools that you're going to use for the rest of your life." If that doesn't work, show them there's superstars doing yoga, relate it to their dreams; for an athlete, show them physical and mental benefits, make it fun, be their friend. Once you make that bond, that friendship, they want to participate, because they know you care.

This level of care and attunement makes HLF's yoga effective as a practice for resilience and unity. Andres and the other teachers at HLF come together with the youth and help the youth bridge various aspects of their lived experience. This is a different approach than a larger yoga studio, where someone may not even know your name let alone your dreams and the role that yoga plays in that.

Andres emphasizes that the *practice* of yoga is the important thing; the effects are going to happen, but we cannot be attached to what they are or what they should be. "Things like employability [and] building of community are byproducts. When we went inward ourselves, doing the process on ourselves, and saw the transformation within us, we thought we'd be remiss to not spread that around [to] others [who are] suffering. Come to people in a very practical way. Do the practice, on yourself, and do the work, don't look for results. Show neighbors, families, friends."

Welcoming in new energy, practices, and knowledge from the ever-growing community of participants in the organization has allowed each organization to gain more trust from their community. These organizations specifically listen to people on the margins—people who are trans, fat, disabled, immigrants, and/or people of color—seeing their lived experience as essential knowledge to tap in to in order to make the organization stronger and more relevant. These organizations have been led by members of these very communities since the beginning, so it's not an add-on that the organization takes on diversity, equity, and inclusion work. In an ongoing way for each organization, justice is a practice.

Nikki Myers reflected on how she incorporates the teachings of yoga into the very functioning of Y12SR with this example: "We used to call the breath guide the 'breath diva' or the 'breath dude.' At some point, the organization as a whole became much more aware that none of that should be gender specific. It was being nonattached to a policy or point of view; the nonattachment philosophy of the organization allows ease of flow or ease of change. If we're really living nonattachment, then that flexibility is possible." The yogic philosophy of nonattachment (Aparigraha) allows the organization to shift and grow as needed. The staff and teachers of Y12SR call upon their practice rather than remaining steadfast in the way that they have always done something or going into a shame spiral because they didn't have a gender-expansive name for the breath guide to begin with. Their practice allows them to look honestly at their reinstatement of the gender binary, to let it go, and to shift to ultimately be more in alignment with the organization's values.

Brenda Salgado expressed gratitude for EBMC's founding teachers and their dedication to the continuing process of creating a teaching faculty that provided safety for marginalized members of society and upheld the organization's values of anti-oppression and inclusivity. In a moment when the attendance of people of color was shifting, EBMC held a community listening circle, where sangha members shared that one teacher, Mushim Patricia Ikeda, consistently read multicultural agreements and created safety, but some other teachers did not. The staff decided that the agreements should be posted on the wall and visible to the sangha to reference during weekly sits or retreats. EBMC teachers would be trained to work with these agreements and encouraged to revisit the agreements that they made regularly, so that they're not just signed and filed away. Brenda reflected that this also led to the requirement that people in teaching roles at EBMC have a set of specific skills that are rarely required at other sanghas, relating to anti-oppression and centering those most targeted. She stated, "If they're not of value to you, it's not that you're good or bad, but just that you're not a good fit. It's not just that we are teaching, we are also teachable, and have some humility about [where we are unaware]. Welcoming is about tapping into the wisdom the community has to make this a better place. There is a lot of wisdom from the margins. It may be different models and structures than you're used to." Some of the core competencies at EBMC include reviewing the community agreements at the beginning of each meditation, workshop, or retreat; acknowledging different realities of participants due to privilege and oppression; making the space accessible to people of various disabilities; and being fragrance free.[2] The teachers are approved by EBMC's board of directors and are periodically reviewed by "lay" or nonteaching members of the board; they are also not assumed to have the answers to all community conflicts that may arise just because they are teachers.[3]

Andres insisted that the continual practice of yoga is the most important thing. "We embody the practice. All [three co-founders] meditate. When our staff tell us they're going through something, their parent said this, frustrated with their job, we ask them, have you meditated? They look at us like, 'Man, come on.' If we didn't get in our sitting time, I would go bonkers and crazy, and that's a huge part of why we are so conscious, and grounded. Our emotions and frustrations are there, but they don't come through as much because we are even-keeled. We can see it through with a different kind of lens." Through this modeling, the three co-founders firmly ingrain the practice in their community.

The organizational practice of being led by practice is something that all of these organizations have in common, and it turns "organizational development" or "strategic planning" on its head, suggesting that we observe where the practice is taking us and direct an organization's strategy based on those observations rather than planting a five- or ten-year strategic plan on the organization and continually building toward that. Their practice leads them into what adrienne maree brown coined as an "emergent strategy."[4]

Community-Led Direction/Community Impact

These organizations have been around to see the results of their offering. Holistic Life Foundation has existed since 2001, Y12SR since 2004, and EBMC since 2007. Each organization has cared for and been shaped by their community. For many yoga and dharma practitioners in general, difficulty brings us to the practice—personal difficulty, like divorce, death of loved ones, and transitions in employment or family life, and also greater systemic oppression that has touched our lives, such as gun violence, poverty, and sexual violence. In projects that specifically orient to suffering, like addiction, in the case of Y12SR, or root themselves in targeted communities, as EBMC and HLF have done, the vulnerability and the potential impact are significant. Brenda shares that over the years, "EBMC helped people through great suffering—breakups, depression and suicide, loss of relationship or family member, coming out. In dark moments, individuals heard from their supporters to go to EBMC, which then became a lifeline, allowing them to feel and be with those things, but that it's okay to put them down as well, to release them after you acknowledge them."

Yoga has assisted the youth involved with HLF in having self-determined, self-empowered lives; it has helped them to be self-regulated in the midst of the conditions of their community, neglected by city and state programs and targeted by police violence. HLF's programs have resulted in higher graduation rates, decreased detention and suspension rates, and increased employment rates after high school graduation. Because they were one of the earlier programs to be offered consistently in public schools, data collected on their programs provide some of the longest-standing evidence in the field of yoga and mindfulness in schools. "Some of [the effect of yoga] is how they handle themselves, where they are not fighting as much, being as disruptive," says Andres. "A lot of it is seeing them acting different in their neighborhood. You can see them do that pause, take a breath, and they don't punch the kid. Some stay through high school, but a lot drop out of our programs—they're involved in sports, girlfriends, boyfriends. [In] high school we lose them a little. When they come back, they always say how much difference we make—a lot of it is with the breath. Helps them focus, relax. They take on the practice themselves, use the tools we gave them in some way, shape, or form."

Nikki described a similar impact of the breath on a young mother who had been attending Y12SR for six months: "[She] was on a work release program, had gotten her kids back from Child Protective Services, and had a really bad day. She used the tools of Y12SR, said, 'I felt this anger and rage that was in my body'—so she recognized what was going on at the level of her body. 'It was coming up through me, and then I paused and heard this voice, which said, "Let's just root and ground and take a deep breath with Mary Jo."' So I took a breath and I didn't beat my kid." Nikki's student chose a different neural pathway, rather than the pattern previously established in her life, what yogis call a *samskara*. These little moments can shift the trajectory of our days, our relationships, our work, and our presence in the world. In these moments we practice yoga—the breath, the self-regulation, the awareness of our sensations, emotions, and postures in any given daily moment. A profound difference between yoga service organizations and yoga studios is this instruction and reflection from participants that the practice of yoga doesn't end once they roll up their mats. In a grand sense, that is where their yoga practice begins. Nikki continued, "My hope is that looking at addiction as a whole, sooner or later, you have to get to how you process reality. When I do that from a yogic perspective, I'm getting at *avidya*. My hope and prayer is that Y12SR grows into a way, a mechanism to look at far more than a substance or a process, but to look at how we view our reality." *Avidya* is a Sanskrit word meaning ignorance, or a lack of wisdom or experience; one of the aspirations as yogis is to cross from ignorance into understanding, from avidya to vidya.

Each organization hires students and graduates as staff and leaders—people who have been transformed by the practices. Brenda reflected further, "During the time I was director, I was excited that our community members would express a desire to build a community library, or a bike rack. The founders of EBMC have always believed in lifting up and encouraging community leadership. It is important to support ideas arising out of the sangha. People would say, 'That's why I give back, it's my place, it's special, we help to shape things, it's not something you're doing to us or for us, but we're building it together.'" In this way, each of these organizations are not about a singular charismatic leader (though their leaders are indeed charismatic!) but about building a community of practice, participation, empowerment, and generosity.

Resistance/Struggles

Andres Gonzalez, Nikki Myers, and Brenda Salgado each spoke of resistance that they meet teaching—whether it's the parameters around teaching yoga in schools, the difficulty in getting into prisons, negotiating gentrification and increased police presence, or navigating the world of addiction recovery that largely doesn't touch embodiment. Indeed, we are creating new work in the world and will come up against the old guard, the mainstream, and what is considered the norm; we each know that this mainstream and norm are inherently harmful and must be shifted. We do this work grounded in our practice, which connects us to a greater wisdom and perspective and nourishes us to keep doing the work of building bridges and creating vitality for all of our communities. Black theologian Ruby Sales suggests that we do this work simultaneously "with a vision of love and a vision of outrage"—outrage at the presence of injustice; love of the dream of justice.[5]

Teaching within institutions, organizations have to be mindful of the policies and practices of the institution and adjust their offerings accordingly, using language that will resonate rather than trigger, offering the purpose of the practice to participants in a transparent way, and thoughtfully considering where the funding comes from and if there is a conflict of interest. When teaching within targeted communities, the organization is affected by what impacts the community—such as gentrification and increased police presence in downtown Oakland, where EBMC is located. Each organization intimately knows the internal and external transformative possibility of the practices, and each grieves their watering down or superficial application.

Andres discussed the challenge of being honest and transparent about HLF's practice while making it palatable in Baltimore public schools: "Our logo is the Om symbol, but instead of the bindu, it's the world. Our logo is even embedded in who we are and what we do. We have to be so careful about the words and terms—we're saying, 'this is stress and relaxation.' We feel like the spiritual aspect of what we believe and what made us who we are, it's missing in what we offer, and we can't teach it in the schools." The separation of church and state arises when teaching yoga in schools, and teachers are required to "secularize" the practice. The benefit of that is that the practice can plant seeds in unexpected or uncommon places; the cost is that some parts of the practice are welcome while others are not. As seen in the 2013 Encinitas School District case that went to the California Supreme Court, a risk of bringing in the "cultural artifacts" of yoga is that the entire program in a school district can be shut down.[6] "Our after-school program has more leeway; we might sneak in a Om chant, a teaser," continues Andres. "If kids are to ask me stuff, I'm more open and willing to say stuff that I wouldn't in the school."

For EBMC, gentrification is a grave concern, threatening to displace the community that the organization serves. Brenda reflected,

> *Our mission is to serve a certain set of community. It may be possible that in three years we need to move because those we want to serve won't be here anymore. Wealthy white technology folks are moving in, and it may be that we need to move to East Oakland or Richmond. Already people who live in the neighborhood who are low income are seeing more police presence—technology people cross the street, clutch their purse—not feeling safe in the neighborhoods that they've lived in for decades. Cops are called for drums in the park by the lake, or during choir practice. People are moving in and being judgmental*

about cultural and racial practices that have been there forever. There is a feeling of unsafety here in downtown Oakland, of not being welcome where you've lived your whole life. Rent control buildings are being neglected, people leave or transition out due to aging, and then they can demolish the building and build a new thing that is not conditioned by rent control. We are hearing from so many activists about being pushed out.

Y12SR has faced challenges within the larger yoga world as well as within addiction and recovery circles. Nikki described the resistance from the mainstream yoga world to discussing addiction as "a superficial kind of 'why would I want to admit the dark side; we're all light, we're all wonderful,'" or from the realm of recovery, "The notion that changing how I hold my body in space really has any kind of effect on character or anything is unaccepted."

The misunderstanding or misapplication of the practice is another worry of the leaders of these practices, and they fear that those errors will be passed down from teacher to student. They each cited class dynamics surrounding yoga and Buddhism—the cost impacts who can actually be in the room. Nikki shared her thoughts about the mainstream yoga world: "I'm grateful that yoga is getting the exposure that it's getting. I get sad dened by the watering down. There's something that knocks my gut and my heart when I see yoga philosophy misused or applied in an individualistic, separate way. There is a piece of that in the trendy commercialism of it." Andres agrees, saying, "I call it Hollywood Hatha. We're doing stuff for people who can't afford that stuff. Even when we go to Omega [in Rhinebeck, New York], they ask us, 'Do you see it getting more diverse?' We say, 'No! It's too expensive. If you want other people to come here, you have to level those prices.' It seems like they don't want to get to those neighborhoods where I'm working. It has to be offered for free to get the buy-in, then maybe, eventually, they'll pay."

Love/Liberation

In speaking to each of these leaders, I was moved by the love that guides them and their organizations. It is a love that is both humble and fierce, gentle and determined, attentive and spacious. None of these leaders have anything to prove; they are not motivated by fame, notoriety, or reputation, yet due to their relentless kindness, innovation, and integrity, they inevitably gain these things. As I know from my own work and that of many healing justice organizations, the practice is to keep showing up, both when it is hard and the world is falling apart and amid celebration. Each organization is invested in individual and collective change—not one without the other—and devotes the appropriate time to that as they grow trust.

EBMC replaces the term *sit* with *meditate* so that people of all bodies feel welcome into practice, whatever the state of their body. "What other center thinks of that?" asked one participant. "It sounds small, but there's a bit of dignity restored when I feel seen like that."[7] EBMC has many practices, informed by its community, that center people who are otherwise marginalized or targeted—a beautiful manifestation of lovingkindness. Another participant reflected in *Lion's Roar* magazine, "To have a radical acceptance for individuals, no matter what, is the work the EBMC is doing and doing well, while making mistakes and learning from those mistakes, and figuring out how to move forward in such a way as to hold that responsibility with tenderness."[8]

I asked Nikki about what it means to be a Y12SR teacher specifically, or to be recognized or take the seat of a teacher more broadly—how to be accountable to the power involved and not get swept up in it. She said, "The training itself is all about a reflection for Y12SR leaders—for space holders to see that it's not really about the other person at all. You're not really going out there to be the savior or to help anybody, to quote Lilla Watson. I read her quote in the training, and I say, if you get this, then I've done my job. Self-reflection in any moment when a space holder is guiding a class—that is a process of reflection, that everyone's liberation is bound together." Nikki insists that it's not about the leader but about self-reflection and continued growth. In doing this, her own "flaws" or mistakes become a teaching tool, not an obstacle or source of shame. Confronted with an error or misstep, she humbly looks inward to reflect on what is true, and then the doorway to gratitude opens: this is an opportunity to grow.

Andres says, "We did it all ourselves, saw what it did to us, and we wanted to spread it. The love just takes over. I know that I am you and you are me. When you get that awareness, it makes you just want to love everyone and everything and figure out how." That insight into interdependence, that I am you and you are me, is a practice of justice and love—for if I am you and you are me, I can't exploit your community for cheap labor, or pollute your water or not intervene in food deserts. Andres's determination to "figure out how" to befriend all people means that he and the greater organization are forging relationships with people in their community who are alike and different, who are visible and invisible. What I have seen from these projects is that they don't give up on anyone, because to do so is to give up on our own selves and our collective potential. They keep offering up the practices to resistant teenagers and reluctant families, continually planting the seeds of practice, and when something sprouts they cultivate it, whether that is through working with parents, starting a new program at a new school, or supporting their participants through individual and collective tragedy with specific practices.

My hope in writing about these organizations is to provide a model of what yoga and meditation *can* look like, what it *is* looking like, outside of and challenging to the mainstream and status quo. These organizations are using the practices to evolve humanity, rather than using them to evade our greatest problems. They are deeply devoted to individual and collective liberation, taking the time, confronting injustice, and building the relationships that allow human creativity to flourish.

Perhaps you see some of your own projects and organizations in them. Perhaps you know about mistakes and gaps that I did not write about. Again, like the rest of us, they are imperfect and brilliant.[9]

TEACHING QUEER
AND TRANS YOGA

"WHY DO LGBTQ people need a separate space, a separate class—isn't that exclusive?" People have asked me this question over fifteen years of teaching Queer and Trans Yoga. My answer is that the class is needed now, given oppression within and beyond yoga in the US. Ultimately, I would love every yoga class to truly embrace all students, of every gender, ability, race, and age. That is just not the case right now. Until we take on oppression and privilege and its dynamics in yoga classrooms, trainings, and retreats, a class like Queer and Trans Yoga is needed to provide queer and trans people with the lifesaving tools and skills of yoga.

Queer and trans students report seeking refuge in the teachings and teachers, only to experience further homophobia, heterosexism, racism, transphobia, fatphobia, and ableism. Likewise, I have begun teaching a Baby & Me class that is attended not exclusively but predominantly by queer families, and I have begun teaching Prenatal Queer and Trans Yoga as well, given my experience in the birthing world. Every Body Yoga and Buddha Body Yoga exist for fat people and Brown Sugar Yoga and POC Yoga exist for folks of color. I hope that this is no longer needed at some point, but until we practice equity and justice as a greater "yoga community," affinity spaces are absolutely vital to marginalized folks practicing at all.

Queer and Trans Yoga and Trauma

Yoga teacher Calia Marshall reflected once, "There's so much pain that comes with trying to be who you are in a society that doesn't approve of who you are." Society is constantly telling queer and trans people that we shouldn't exist, through overt and subversive forms of oppression. When we do not possess the tools and presence to shield ourselves from or uproot these continuous messages, we experience trauma that embeds itself in our bodies and hearts, our relationships, and our community.

In the summer of 2012 in Brooklyn, three trans people in our community took their own lives; every year we lose more of our kindred. Reported murders of trans women of color continue to increase, and because they are underreported and underinvestigated and victims' gender identities are not always identified correctly, these rates may be much higher than what is reported.[1] In 2016, over two hundred anti-LGBTQ bills were introduced to state legislatures, and a mass shooting took place at Pulse, a gay nightclub in Orlando, Florida. I write about trauma because amid all of our fabulousness, our role in social change, and the incredible art that queer and trans people contribute to the world, there is a shadow side, the effect of insidious trauma, the trauma of oppression. I recognize that this is not unique to the queer community, or to my queer community; any community that faces oppression faces trauma in the body, heart, mind, spirit, and sangha.

The offering of Queer and Trans Yoga recognizes the existence and persistence of trauma among queer and trans people—trauma to the individual, which varies among individuals, and the trauma that we collectively hold. This includes suicides; harassment and assault; murder; denial of services, employment, education, and housing; and high rates of incarceration. Risk of trauma is higher for those of us who are queer and/or trans and also disabled, elders, youth, immigrants, formerly incarcerated, or have other overlapping marginalized experiences. In a post for the blog Black Girl Dangerous, Travis Alabanza wrote, "White definitions about how to deal with trauma are steeped in the privileged assumption that you have been told by the world that you are fully human. That you have been told that you can heal, can hurt and can access help. As a Black Queer person living under these oppressive systems, that is not something I have been told. Before I could begin to heal, I had to learn to access the humanity I had been denied under these systems."[2] This discrimination exists, and we hold both this history and current reality in our individual bodies, hearts, and souls, and collectively as a queer sangha.

The practice of yoga encourages us to examine our behaviors and look deeply into them—do they come from a place of fear, or even terror? In class we can examine our experiences of trauma and how they affect every-day thinking, emotional responses, and embodiment. We can anticipate a trigger, and use resources of breath, sensation, and orienting to the space that we're in to keep us in the here and now, so that we might respond to a difficult moment or situation in a way that is healing.

We seek practices that ground, heal, and self-regulate us. This is an act of self-love and community love that creates resilience. Larry Yang offers,

> One of the characteristics embedded in Mindfulness is the capacity to remem-ber that our personal and collective Freedom is not dependent on any external conditions. Justice, as worthy a task as it is in our lives, will take longer to fulfill than any of us would like. It will require the efforts of the many rather than the few. And it will require every spiritual attribute and resource we can muster. There is tremendous injustice and unfairness in our cultures, our society, and our world. And our Freedom is not even dependent upon Life being fair or just. True Freedom does not mean to be in a place where there is no problem, struggle, or oppression. True Freedom means to be in the midst of those things, and still have clarity in our minds, openness in our hearts, and integrity in our actions. This is the kind of Freedom that will allow us to move through even our most difficult struggles with greater effectiveness, ease, and benefit for us all.[3]

Healing trauma does not necessitate an end to injustices, but rather pro-vides us with tools to be present and skillful in the midst of injustices, neu-tral circumstances, and pleasures. Of course we seek to create a just society, but as Larry Yang suggests, that road is long. In the meantime, yoga and mindfulness practices prevent us from perpetuating further harm out of our own dysregulation.

Students in my Queer and Trans Yoga classes often have not other-wise had the opportunity to be in their bodies as their whole selves. I have worked with trans people who have been hiding their chests and shrinking their presence to avoid harassment, to avoid being seen by cruel eyes. I have worked with countless couples going through a breakup in a small community. I have worked with cisgender men uprooting patriarchal patterns within them. I have worked with trans people who were harassed on the train on the way to class. I have worked with gender nonconforming people with such unique style and presence in the world, one of whom told me, "I tried to sequester my fashion, my style, and it almost killed me. So now I let it live, let it shine, and hope for the best."

An important aspect of affinity classes is mirroring. Children need mirroring for their own psychological development, and marginalized people need it as well. People with privilege receive consistent mirroring—seeing themselves reflected in history books, media, advertising. As Travis Alabanza asks as a queer Black person, "How could I know I could heal, if I had never been shown that people with my identities even experienced trauma?"[4] It is important not just that queer and trans people access yoga, meditation, and other healing practices but also that we be held by community leaders who have healed themselves, too. Having a teacher and sangha reflect back to us various aspects of ourselves is as important as the science of the practice itself.

Yoga teacher and queer Israeli Danny Arguetty describes the physical and energetic imprint of trauma as follows: "If the flow of breath, and thus prana, through both our gross and subtle realms is hindered or decreased, we ultimately spend more time in a contracted state of being. This physical and energetic shift, which often results from a learned pattern of holding, can eventually lead to a profound sense of isolation and separateness. Conversely, the more we nurture the breath body, the more sensitive we become to our internal and external worlds; from this space of attunement, we are better equipped to make conscious, empowered decisions in life."[5] The cultivation of the breath is healing and empowering from the inside out, as we protect and nurture the breath through toning our physical bodies and surrounding ourselves with people and environments that nourish us, and from that place of groundedness and wholeness, we can be more effective in encountering and transforming what is ungrounded and broken in the world.

We hold so many stories, so much history, as a community—both current and past circumstances for queer and trans people in the world. Queer and trans people get killed every day. We get ostracized from our families of origin. We lose jobs for being who we are. We are at greater risk for suicide and greater risk of assault. We are surveilled by police—more or less so depending on the color of our skin. We may be wrongly gendered in prisons, homeless shelters, domestic violence shelters, and immigration detention shelters, and we have a bigger fight to face than our straight and cisgender peers in similar circumstances. And we hear about these stories every day, as that is the lived reality of our lovers, friends, coworkers, families. Of course, for queer and trans folks of color, these realities are even more grave.

It can be a lot to hold all these truths and realities in our own lives and that of those around us and close to us—we can become overwhelmed. Having a yoga or meditation practice can expand the presence that holds those difficulties. When a teaspoon of salt is put into a cup of water, the water may taste quite salty. However, when a teaspoon of salt is deposited into a barrel of water, we may not be able to taste that salt at all. That is what our practice does—it creates expansion and spaciousness, which leads to resilience.

Queer Folks, Trauma, and Addiction

The source of our trauma is ultimately injustice, oppression, colonization, and capitalism. Addiction is a result of the trauma of injustice. Canadian doctor Gabor Maté says, "In large population studies, you find that extreme trauma, whether in a population like the Native Indian population in [the US] or the Aboriginal population in Australia or the Native population in my country with the loss of land and the violence and the forced abduction of their children who were brought up for a hundred years in residential schools away from their families where they were sexually abused, generation after generation, there's a huge statistical and causative link between that trauma and the addiction. That's not a theory. It's just reality."[6] I find this empowering—a missing link between injustice, activism, and healing. If we don't (or cannot) heal the source of our trauma, we attempt to manage its effects on ourselves with coping mechanisms such as addiction. If we are only addressing the source of our trauma through activism, artistic expression, or education, but not healing our bodies, hearts, and minds, then we inevitably recreate the trauma in our lives.

Queer folks are more likely to have experienced trauma, we face high rates of depression connected to homophobia and heterosexism in our world, and we often struggle to find our place in the world, experiencing high levels of stress, so it's no wonder that studies have found that lesbian, gay, and bisexual people are twice as likely to have an addiction than our straight counterparts.[7] LGBTQ youth are more than two times as likely to be bullied, assaulted, or excluded at school and almost half less likely than non-LGBTQ youth to have a reliable, supportive adult to whom they can turn.[8] Additionally, there is a party culture in queer community, which can normalize the use of substances and increases the risk of addiction.

When queer folks do seek help, we often encounter homophobia in addiction treatment facilities. Interestingly, when you do a Google search for queer people and addiction, pages upon pages come up, many of them redirecting you to drug treatment facilities that have no specific practices for working with LGBTQ people or discrimination or harassment protection for the individuals in treatment. Canada's Substance Abuse and Mental Health Services Administration explains, "The reasons LGBT individuals may avoid or delay seeking professional care include fear of disclosing their sexual orientation or gender and previous experiences with health-care providers who attempted to convert them to heterosexuality, who attributed their substance abuse to their sexual or gender orientation, or who were otherwise judgmental and unsupportive."[9] A 2020 study through New York University showed that lesbian, gay, and bisexual older adults are more likely than their straight counterparts to use substances, likely in part as a way of coping with homophobia and heterosexism over the course of their lives. "Even though times are changing and things have been getting better for the LGBTQ community, older individuals in this population may still be affected from past experiences of intolerance," said researcher Joseph Palamar, associate professor in the Department of Population Health at NYU Langone Health.[10]

Queer communities are hurting from the experience of homophobia, heterosexism, and transphobia, and we need practices to heal and healers to hold us through it. Gabor Maté reflects, "Addiction is a response to suffering. You're not going to make people give up addiction by making them suffer more."[11] Queer healers and allies working with queer communities are entrusted with this work of harm reduction and societal healing. It's not enough to treat the individual when the source of the wound continues. Our healers must also be working for a world of justice. We must provide our communities with healthier tools to cope with the immediate impact of trauma (such as mindfulness, yoga, dance, and prayer), strive to overthrow or dismantle the systems of oppression that create that trauma in the first place, and integrate self-care and community care in our homes, businesses, organizations, and neighborhoods.

Queer Resilience

Vicarious resilience is another reason to teach or attend a class like Queer and Trans Yoga for a specific community with common experiences: through being around one another, and witnessing each other's laughter, joy, tears, vulnerability, and strength, we relate to and internalize nobility and vulnerability as a community. We internalize the power, fortitude, and vitality from our community from being around it, from being mirrored, through witnessing struggles, growth, and transformation. In Queer and Trans Yoga, we connect with our growth, pain, and resilience, and recognize our human capacity to thrive. Each time we show up to this class, we are expressing gratitude for our own lives and that of one another. In a community that copes with high rates of suicide, harassment, murder, and other forms of trauma, showing up to be present with each other is extremely important. Becky Thompson writes in *Survivors on the Yoga Mat*, "Prana can be collectively produced—the more people there are to generate the prana, the more of it there is, and the more likely it is that others will keep joining in. Prana is electric; it wires us all together. Prana is like an energetic form of serotonin, a natural caffeine. Everybody could use exposure to this 'drug,' perhaps trauma survivors especially, because prana carries hope."[12]

This is the value of practicing together, of joining in sangha, or blessed community. There is an energy created in the room, called *prana* in Sanskrit. Yet, when the dynamics of oppression are recycled in mindfulness spaces, it's very difficult for targeted and marginalized practitioners to remain present and open, for the place we come to seek solace is a place that recreates the very harms we are trying to heal. This is the importance of specialized classes, for there is less likelihood of fatphobia, racism, misogyny, and transphobia being recreated, and there is a community container for when they are. We seek a balance between accessing a "safer space" and surrendering to the reality of dukkha, that suffering exists in the world and will continue to exist in our lives. When our practice is strong enough to withstand the microaggressions, we can access more generalized classes, because the dukkha doesn't hurt so much because we have begun to heal our wounds. Then we can access the collective prana that Becky Thompson writes of, across all kinds of difference.

Tools in Teaching Queer and Trans Yoga

I teach Queer and Trans Yoga no differently than I teach any other yoga class, and the context for our practice is specific. There are jokes or reference points that we hold as a community, and some poses, like Crane Pose, do have a particular gay aesthetic; occasionally during a lovingkindness meditation I ask the students to have a particular focus on queer community, offering our love to queer elders, to queer people we know of but do not know personally, and to people whom we have difficulty with in the moment. This would be the case in any community or specialized class, like a prenatal class or a class for cancer survivors. Thus, the context for the class is different than a general yoga class.

Queer and Trans Yoga allows more room for gender and varied ways of loving and creating family. As a queer and trans yoga teacher, these are approaches that I utilize regardless of whether I am teaching a Queer and Trans Yoga class that arise out of my own experience of feeling hurt, dismissed, or disregarded in yoga classes—I use those experiences to be extra kind, mindful, and engaged with my students. Part of the intention in teaching Queer and Trans Yoga is a recognition that transphobia, homophobia, and heterosexism exist, intertwined with other forms of oppression. They exist within all of us, within every space that we create, and they are perpetuated if we are not mindful of our thoughts, words, and deeds. Thus, at the center of how I teach is holding space for the pain and scars that oppression has created, as well as a belief in and affirmation of our resilience, importance, and fabulousness.

There are specific understandings and practices that teachers can cultivate that allow one to be an ally to queer and trans people that I share below. These are just some tools; more exist, this list is incomplete. I invite you to try them on, and continue expanding from here.

Gendered Language

I do not use gendered language in any classes, which I hear in almost every other yoga class I attend. This means phrases like "this is a good pose for women," or "if you are a man, lay your hands in your lap with the left hand on top of the right," or "men may find this pose easier than women." When such language is used in classes, queer and trans folks may feel left out, unacknowledged, and dismissed. I speak more specifically about energetics that I think these comments are trying to address, such as, "If you are needing more vigor today, do X; if you are needing more tenderness, do Y." This allows the humanity of each student, no matter their sexuality or gender, to be more fully expressed.

Queer Realities and Contexts

I teach asana, philosophy, meditation, and breathwork in a Queer and Trans Yoga class, but the context, the embodied and political experience of students and the community already created before we enter the room, is different. This would be the case for any class for a specific community—such as disabled people, fat folks, or people of color. Part of being a community is having common experience, reference points, and culture, and in Queer and Trans Yoga class, we celebrate ourselves and mourn our losses together.

Since students present have experiences of homophobia, misogyny, and transphobia, I speak to that in my Queer and Trans Yoga classes. When we are practicing karuna (compassion) meditation I might ask my students to aspire toward offering karuna to their harasser, the boss who just fired them for being queer, or their ex-lover. When we are folding forward, I might speak to bowing to our queer and trans selves and all that that identity entails or brings forth. When we are in *Savasana* (Relaxation Pose), trying to let go, I might speak of letting go of shame, of guilt, of shields that we may hold in our bodies, hearts, and minds.

Queering Yoga Gear

A difference that I see in my Queer and Trans Yoga classes, workshops, and retreats is what people wear. This may seem to be a trivial difference, but it can make someone immediately comfortable or uncomfortable, like they fit in or that they don't belong; it is one of the first things we often notice in walking into a space. The "yoga chic" aesthetic can be a straight and cisgender aesthetic, although there is a way for many of us to queer it up. That clothing line is not usually one that many Queer and Trans Yoga students are aware of, interested in, or financially able to access, for this class is often their first time practicing yoga in a studio setting. What queer and trans students wear to class can vary, for I have seen tweed sports coats, basketball shorts, political T-shirts, jeans, sequins, and scrubs. What I love about the queering of yoga gear is that it makes much more room for practitioners from other communities, making the practice seem more accessible to a wider swath of humanity.

Bring on the Sass

My Queer and Trans Yoga students often talk back, groan, and otherwise express themselves more than students in a typical class. I think that this is because of the culture of most yoga classes, and the value that queer culture has in being expressive. I'll bring my students into *Utkatasana* (Chair Pose) for a fifth time, and they'll do it, but say, "Oh no you di'int!" or I'll put them in Downward-Facing Dog *(Adho Mukha Svanasana)* for the first time, and they'll say, "Are you for real? This is a pose?" or they'll be in plank for up to a minute, and they'll say, "Is this over yet?" They will sing along with songs; they will groan when it gets hard and sigh when they get relief. People in the room may break into vogueing, as often happens when I work with queer youth especially! I encourage vocalization in my general population classes, but those are rarely as talkative as even the quietest Queer and Trans Yoga class.

Queer Is Political

As discussed earlier, *queer* is more than a sexual orientation; it is a political identity, and most people who are specifically queer-identified have a progressive, anti-oppressive politic about them. Thus, I can talk about Black Lives Matter in my Queer and Trans Yoga classes, talk about grief after the killings at the Charleston AME church, and reference the presidential campaign of Bernie Sanders. I wear political T-shirts when I teach without fear of offending or alienating someone. In general yoga classes, I try to have my reference points be love, kindness, and integrity, with the goal of welcoming everyone into the practice and meeting my students where they are at. In a Queer and Trans Yoga class, it's a more specific, smaller swath of society, and one that I am greatly familiar with. I make connections between the dharma and political events in Queer and Trans Yoga, using the events themselves as a teaching.

That Sounds Queer

The music that I play in Queer and Trans Yoga classes can also differ from that of my other classes. I often try to have most musicians in a given playlist be queer-identified, and include various queer cultural icons such as Barbra Streisand, Antony and the Johnsons, Madonna, David Bowie, Beyoncé, and Adele. I have specific playlists for Queer and Trans Yoga classes and workshops.

I once taught a Queer and Trans Yoga class for Aspen Gay Ski Week, an annual event in Aspen, Colorado, but due to the studio's misunderstanding and inaccurate marketing, none of the students who attended were queer and didn't know it was a queer and trans–specific yoga class. I had prepared a wonderful playlist of queer musicians and queer icons, and I still played the playlist, but it did not resonate as it would have for queer and trans students—no one sang along or giggled, as is often the case in my Queer and Trans Yoga classes when students recognize the cultural significance of a song or hear the lyrics of a song validate a core part of their queer or trans experience.

Trauma-Informed Teaching

Many people within queer communities are survivors of sexual violence—64 percent of trans people, 13 percent of lesbians, half of bisexual men and women, and 40 percent of gay men.[13] To "be in the body" can feel quite dangerous, for the body has been a site of harm, and a survival mechanism can be dissociation, when our attention leaves the body. Some queer and trans folks have been targeted by homophobic and transphobic violence. For trans people, our bodies haven't necessarily resonated with our identities or internal experiences of ourselves; to be told or invited to "be in the body" when our bodies don't feel quite our own can feel naïve or cruel.

I speak directly to the experience of trauma in class and share that safety in our bodies is not a given, not an arrival point, but rather a process. I try to destigmatize trauma—there can be an idea that part of what made us queer or trans is this trauma; overcoming the shame of trauma is mixed with internalized homophobia and transphobia. I welcome students to not practice what I'm teaching but to feel empowered to move on their own, and I provide space for self-practice for everyone. I allow space for breakdowns, and we hold them as a community. I teach my students resources for staying in the moment—being aware of breath and sensation, orienting to the space that they're in—so that they become aware of time-traveling back to times and sites of trauma and differentiate the present moment from previous experiences.

~≈

In the yoga classroom, we can lean on the teachings of yoga as a source of strength, as well as each other's life paths and experiences. We co-regulate together—when someone's breath is deep, facial expressions are welcoming, and voice is calm, then it helps everyone around that person be emotionally regulated as well. Thus, in Queer and Trans Yoga, we are learning tools to be emotionally regulated through the practice of yoga and growing stronger as a community as we build off of each other's vitality and resilience. We learn about each other's methods of resilience and vitality and the ways that we internalize some of the hate in the world around us. I work to hold space for the difficulty, celebrate the resiliency, and make room for everything in between.

INJUSTICE PRODUCES TRAUMA; HEALING CREATES CONDITIONS FOR JUSTICE

TRAUMA IS ONE of those words that has entered the popular lexicon in recent years and is often used incorrectly. Trauma does not stand in for something that is difficult; something can be difficult and yet not cause trauma. Trauma is something that overwhelms your ability to cope, leaving you feeling helpless, hopeless, and out of control. Our mechanisms for dealing with any difficult situation are fight, flight, freeze, or appease; when these strategies do not work, that is the experience of trauma. When we are unable to fight off danger, unable to freeze until something leaves us alone and we are safe, unable to run away from gunshots, trauma is created. If we have the resources to be with a difficult situation—if we are grounded, present, connected to community, and connected to our bodies in present time, trauma is not created. Trauma is created when we are underresourced or when we cannot access our tools—when our capacity to cope is overwhelmed.

When a reaction to something, like someone grabbing your wrist, is profound, it's likely historical—it has a history of trauma to it. This is called a trigger: something that reminds you of something that happened in the past, to which you react in a way that is out of proportion to what occurred and which causes your nervous system to time travel back to that dangerous situation. Triggers can be sounds, objects, people, specific identities of people, places—anything that reminds a person of a trauma. Healing a trigger, remaining in the here and now, demands patience, attention, and practice, and I explore tools in the section in this chapter entitled "Healing Trauma, Creating Justice."

The effects of trauma include insomnia, problems concentrating, difficulty calming down, poor relationships with others, under- and over-engagement of the nervous system, avoidance, feeling a lack of control, and dissociation. Yoga therapist David Emerson writes, "Trauma has a deep and long-lasting effect on the entire organism, from chemical and anatomical changes in the brain, to changes in our body's physiological systems, to the subjective impact on the experience of the survivor. We believe that treatment for trauma must be equally thorough—considering the person as a whole and addressing the broad-ranging effects of trauma on an individual."[1] Thus, practices that work on the energetic, mental, emotional, and somatic levels can be incredibly impactful in healing trauma.

We're shaped by the big traumas and the little ones. When we don't have tools and resources to deal with traumatic events, they impact our bodies. When we're not able to get ourselves to safety or say what we need to say, trauma energy gets stuck in the body. Tara Brach says, "Traumatic abuse causes lasting changes in our physiology, nervous system and brain chemistry. In the course of normal development, memories are consolidated as we evaluate each new situation in terms of the cohesive worldview we have previously formulated. When there has been trauma, this cognitive process is short-circuited by the surge of painful and intense stimulation."[2] Trauma has many forms; it can be caused by physically terrible events such as accidents, violence, or natural disasters and also emotional experiences such as neglect or mental abuse. Ancestral trauma is another important area of trauma to consider; the experiences of one's ancestors, if not processed and healed, are passed on. It doesn't matter if we know our ancestors' stories of what happened—trauma can be passed on through parenting, interactions with conflict, grieving processes, and familial patterns that sometimes are helpful and sometimes compromise our well-being. When those wounds are processed and healed, the scar formed becomes a powerful resource for resilience, strength, creativity, and healing. Tessa Hicks Peterson writes, "Sometimes trauma is 'big' and imposed impersonally (e.g., war, social violence, state-sponsored violence, natural disasters). Other times it occurs on a more intimate scale (e.g., physical, emotional, verbal, or sexual abuse). Often the individual, intimate experience is linked to systemic oppression, as in the case of sexual violence. Some forms of trauma are one-time events with a high negative impact; this is known as 'shock trauma.' By contrast, 'developmental' or 'complex trauma' refers to an ongoing series of traumatic events."[3]

Where we hold tension can tell the story of what our trauma might be—around the shoulders and neck from not being heard or self-expressed, around the belly from feeling disempowered or overpowered, in the hips from sexual trauma. This is the wisdom of the chakras, a connection between our society, body, mind, and soul, which can be quite powerful to explore, especially if you're not consciously aware of your trauma. Anodea Judith shares in her book on the chakras, "Chakras are the organizing centers for the reception, assimilation, and transmission of our life energies. Our chakras, as core centers, form the coordinating network of our complicated body/mind system."[4] The earliest written reference to the chakras is in the Vedas, and they are also mentioned in the Yoga Upanishads and Yoga Sutras of Patanjali. Trauma lives in the body, and through embodiment practices those stories can be unlocked.

People with unhealed trauma will do extreme things to try to feel, or they may cut themselves off from feeling entirely. People might ride motorcycles at breakneck speed, cut themselves, do extreme sports—all in an attempt to come back into the body and present time. Or trauma survivors will avoid feeling anything at all, ever—by using substances (which I wrote about more extensively in the last chapter) or simply leading incredibly busy lives, going from one thing to the next without space to feel.

If we don't heal our trauma, we run on autopilot. At best, we fail to intervene in suffering around us. At worst, we risk passing on our own pain to our families, colleagues, students, spiritual lineages, and neighborhoods. When we heal, we are self-regulated, grounded, centered, in present time and space, and able to respond based on the wisdom of our integrated experiences. When we don't heal, we can be dysregulated, existing in the future with fear and anxiety, or in the past with resentment, rumination, and aggression. We see this in veterans who return home without adequate resources for healing and may abuse their spouses and children. A very high percentage of people who abuse children were sexually abused themselves and never healed from that trauma. As Gabor Maté explains, "We have seen it in Rwanda, we have seen the Americans slaughter half a million Iraqis, we have seen Israelis slaughter Palestinian children, we have seen American soldiers wiping out men, women and children in Vietnam and get away with it, and we see the horrors perpetrated by the Islamic state in the Middle East right now.... If you look at people who are willing to perpetrate such things, you look usually at traumatized people."[5] If we look deeply into the pain, try to meet it with awareness, compassion, and forgiveness, and then act and speak from deep intention of kindness and integrity, we can heal our own trauma and interrupt the patterns of trauma in our communities.

Information about trauma can be very empowering—it can help us to understand our bodies and minds and why they do what they do in the name of survival. For many of my students, this means removing a layer of self-blame, guilt, and shame and understanding that when trauma occurred, they simply lacked the tools to cope. The body did what it did to survive, but it wasn't a long-term solution—long-term, it compromises well-being. With this information about trauma, we are aware of the context of our practices, and the potential impact.

We must beware, however, that the individualism of meditation practices in the West can sometimes perpetuate trauma. Many meditation retreats have an intake form so that teachers can be made aware of what a student may be bringing. Yet many teachers don't have experience with or training on trauma and may not be skillful when it arises. Buddhist teacher and therapist Tara Brach points out,

> *Specific practices to develop compassion cultivate our capacity to hold with kindness painful or intense experiences that are arising within us. Although taught and practiced in groups, these trainings of heart and mind are primarily a solitary, intrapsychic endeavor. Especially when there has been childhood trauma, "going it alone" in this way can be frightening and disorienting. Mindfulness practices can unleash buried emotions that might re-traumatize the unskilled practitioner. Or, rigid and habitual defenses against raw feelings may impede the ability to focus or relax. In either case, meditation feels discouraging or impossible, only deepening a sense of unworthiness.[6]*

Generative Somatics practitioner and therapist David Treleaven concurs, adding, "As trauma-informed practitioners, we need to remember that institutional structures still commonly deny and repress trauma, and ignore or discount survivors.... Our definitions of trauma influence how we treat groups of people—both as a society and as individual practitioners."[Because the incidence of trauma is so high—it is likely to be in our yoga classrooms and meditation retreats—teachers must be trained and prepared for when it arises and have tools to help a survivor navigate and ground again.

Vicarious trauma is the embodied experiencing of other people's trauma as your own. Vicarious trauma is entrenched in many communities that have faced ongoing trauma—either over years, such as suicides among LGBTQ people, or over generations, such as police brutality against communities of color. One may experience vicarious trauma from being in close quarters with folks who are deep in their own trauma—lovers, colleagues, chosen family. People in service industries (health care, social work, welfare, etc.) as well as people trying to change the way things are (government, social justice, human rights work, policy work, etc.) can experience vicarious trauma when work is taken home and they lack adequate tools to process the difficulty they have been entrusted with. In many instances, understaffing and long work hours with not enough time off play a role in vicarious trauma. Those on the front lines need training, support, and time away from the work to not experience vicarious trauma. Among people working to build our compassion, it can be easy to take that pain on as our own, but it's important for our well-being and longevity in the work that we do not.

We can be present to our lived realities and history without experiencing it as vicarious trauma. In working with CISPES, I learned about "historical memory"—the importance of knowing where we've come from and what we've been through as a way to better locate ourselves in the present and look forward into the future. When we acknowledge a difficult history, hold it in community with our tools, and know that our existence and our work grow out of it, it does not retraumatize. I need my yoga and Buddhism practices in order to remain present to the difficulties and travesties that are present in queer communities—the harassment, the homicides, the suicides, the discrimination in housing, health care, education, and employment—without experiencing the stories and data as vicarious trauma. My practice allows me to ground, to find strength, to weep, to rage, to grieve, and then to engage. Jaya Devi's guru, Ma Jaya Sati Bhagavati, used to say that "we must drink as we pour"—that as we serve and engage with the world around us, we need to fill ourselves back up; we need nourishment to continue. To not practice self-care is not only to deplete ourselves but also to deplete the work, to deplete our communities and networks, and to deplete the efforts for change that are necessary in the world.

Vicarious resilience, on the other hand, is resilience that builds within community. We see it in public spaces, such as a subway car when one person gives up a seat for an elder or pregnant woman and other people follow suit, caring for strangers. Vicarious resilience is seen in social movements, which is part of what makes being in the movement so powerful— witnessing you being strong, caring, or courageous makes me stronger, more caring, more courageous. We see vicarious resilience in community spaces, such as at Black Yoga Teachers Alliance conferences or in Queer and Trans Yoga. As a single finger, we are easily broken, but as a fist, we are strong. Vicarious resilience is part of why targeted people build strong communities: our survival depends on it.

Trauma as a Product of Injustice

"We must have healthy individuals working in healthy organizations that are part of healthy communities that create a healthy society," implores my friend and colleague Lisa Garrett, a social justice organizational developer. All of these layers compose the picture of justice, and so each layer must be healthy and functional. If we do not address trauma, it can eat away at organizations from the inside out, and organizations that take on healing work as an essential component of their work are more resilient for it.

We often think of trauma as an experience that solely "victims," survivors, or oppressed peoples experience. But injustice hurts everyone involved, cutting everyone involved off from a component of their humanity. The Buddha said, "In a battle, both the winners and the losers lose."[8]

I hear in mindfulness and yoga circles discussion of "those who need the practice the most," which often implies low-income communities, communities of color, and other communities with high incidences of trauma. While I obviously support these communities accessing and utilizing healing methodologies, I don't believe that the practices are more important or more impactful among certain communities than others. We all need healing, and we all deserve it. Buddhist teacher and entrepreneur Konda Mason claims, "I know that true planetary healing can only happen once we stop living the myth of separation: separation of nations, separation of races, separations of classes, separation from spirit."[9]

In teaching an earth-based meditation once to an online sangha, we repeated the phrases, "I am the earth, the earth is me" and "you are the earth, the earth is you." After teaching this practice once, sangha members shared that when I invited them to consider someone disconnected from the earth they thought of people like Jared Kushner and Jeff Bezos. We reflected afterward how impactful these practices could be for those holding the most power in our world, if they contemplated and acted from their inherent connection, rather than imagined separation.

If we consider that everyone is injured by oppression and that some people benefit from the injustice or oppression, then the door is opened for more healing. Tessa Hicks Peterson reflects,

Intense emotional reactions are expected to arise in this process. Anticipating such reactions and cultivating awareness so that we can bear witness to them as they unfold within ourselves or in others allows us to learn from this dissonance. With critical self-reflection, deep listening and learning from people who hold other perspectives on these topics, people who hold unearned privileges can recognize the ways in which participation in social change work is an act of resistance to the continuation of institutional oppression.[10]

Karishma Kripalani and I wrote in a 2016 anthology, "For many, yoga is a tool to help us better negotiate the acute and chronic trauma experienced in the world. Anxiety, depression, and other PTSD symptoms, both apparent and not, are present in yoga spaces. Research has shown the impact of oppression, microaggressions and race-based stress as trauma. Yoga is, for many, part of a 'therapeutic landscape' and a site for healing. Yet, the terrain is always, already, shaped by dynamics of power and privilege and our experiences in these spaces may be retraumatizing. Thus, social justice work is also trauma work."[11] We need to recognize the violence and harm facing our communities, from bullying, gun violence, police brutality, war, incarceration, poverty, the so-called War on Drugs, unemployment and underemployment, environmental injustice, gentrification, deportation, and more.

For some, it's not possible to live our lives without knowing oppression directly, and so our work is that of discernment: to not continually bombard our hearts and psyches with stories that our people and ancestors have lived, to moderate our consumption of tragic news, dial up self-care practices, and build collective power. For those protected by privilege, our work is to find reputable, consistent sources and to look at the articles, documentaries, and videos of violence and harm, to let it break our hearts, and to redistribute resources to those most impacted. Many of us enter social justice work to heal ourselves, our communities, and the world. Danielle Sered charges, "Because trauma distills down to powerlessness, the opposite of trauma is not help; the opposite of trauma is power. It will therefore be essential that any reallocation of resources is not top-down, but grounded in an ever-increasing accountability on the part of government systems and community leaders to the political power built by those whose lives are at stake in violence and its elimination."[12]

Healing Trauma, Creating Justice

Healing from trauma involves bringing attention to our bodies, particularly our tension and numbness, and building power among those most impacted. Uncovering and healing trauma demands patience and fortitude, and its timeline cannot be predetermined. As we turn toward the pain in our lives, we get closer to our authentic selves, uncovering a truth of the heart. Healing from trauma is not just something that improves our individual lives—helping us sleep better, digest better, find joy in the everyday—although that is wonderful and important. If we want a "better world," a just world, a world of kindness and accountability, then we must look into our experiences of trauma, heal it, organize among those most impacted, and reallocate resources.

If we suppress or ignore trauma, then we fray relationships with one another and we act out through microaggressions or greater forms of harm, whereas healing from trauma can change the trajectory of our families, organizations, communities, and even our society. And conversely, as Tessa Hicks Peterson suggests, "Radical healing reignites practices that reclaim interconnectedness and the relationships we have lost (to ourselves, to our neighbors, to our communities, and to our environment) as a result of the fragmenting impacts of oppression and our country's devotion to individuation. Cultivating a greater sense of accountability and care (for ourselves, for our neighborhoods, for our communities, and for our environment) is inherent to the reclamation of community healing."[13]

We attend to our bodies once we are safe, once our lives and survival are no longer in jeopardy. It's best to do this work when we feel grounded, centered, and resourced, so that we have appropriate nourishment to help us approach the gravity of our trauma. We work to realize that we are lovable and whole, regardless of what may have happened in our individual lives, our family's trajectory, or the actions and legacies of our ancestors. Connection to the body is vital. We cannot be whole without being embodied, which is the wisdom and utility of yoga or any embodied practice.

In short, how does mindfulness help heal trauma?

- It brings us into present time

- Through gentle attention, we feel sensations that might otherwise be overlooked or shut out

- We connect to pain, turn toward it, listen, and allow it to guide us

- We cultivate self-regulation—the skills and awareness to calm and center ourselves, even among difficult situations, in present time

- We practice in sangha—healing happens in community

Self-regulation refers to the practices that we do to keep ourselves healthy and in present time and place. Prayer, dance, theater, art, writing, yoga, Tai

Chi, and Qigong are all forms of self-regulation that move pent-up energy, build positive energy, and cultivate strength. "When we are self-regulated, it impacts those around us since our energies and nervous systems are in resonance with one another. Internal coherence often impacts and results in external and collective coherence."[14]

Hala Khouri teaches about being "resourced"—purposefully using breath, embodiment, and orientation techniques to remain in present time and space. Orientation involves noticing breath, noticing three unique things about the space that you're in, and noticing sensations in the body to stay present and not in the history where something horrendous occurred. Being resourced provides the freedom to distinguish between a trigger and trauma. Being resourced creates safety more often, for when we have the tools to feel what is happening in our bodies, to be present, to ground, we can respond skillfully.

A tool for healing trauma is to study the lives of those who have lived through grave experiences of trauma and nevertheless are leaders. We then realize that healing is possible. Nelson Mandela, Grace Lee Boggs, John Lewis, Ruby Sales, and Harriet Tubman are examples of people who have turned toward their suffering and transformed it into wisdom and leadership. Elisabeth Kübler-Ross says, "The most beautiful people we have known are those who have known defeat, known suffering, known struggle, known loss, and have found their way out of the depths. These persons have an appreciation, a sensitivity, and an understanding of life that fills them with compassion, gentleness, and a deep loving concern. Beautiful people do not just happen."[15] We are not strong, beautiful, passionate, playful, and creative in spite of our trauma, but because we have survived, healed, and lead. Being present with the pain is essential to organizing. We must not just skip ahead to the rally, press release, or conference but slow down, breathe, and feel.

Accountability and Callout Culture

Accountability means a willingness to face an injury and, through our actions, intentionally heal, whether on an individual or community level. Turning toward the shadows and difficulty is essential in the pursuit of liberation. Individually, we examine our wounds, unskillful patterns, and unwholesome practices, for "what we resist persists" as the aphorism goes. Desmond Tutu and Mpho Tutu van Furth suggest, "If we want real forgiveness and real healing, we must face the real injury."[16]

When we understand that "hurt people hurt people," the healing of wealthy people, men, white people, and others with privilege is absolutely necessary, alongside those in positions of privilege reckoning with the wreckage caused in its wake. Patrisse Cullors reflects, "I remember specifically after the acquittal of George Zimmerman how many anti-racist white folks wrote stories about their own whiteness and their relationship to it. And it was this powerful conversation with the public in this vulnerable way around how people are continually behaving and supporting anti-Black racism by their own behavior. And when Mike Brown was murdered, we saw another round where whole communities, non-Black [people of color] communities in particular, [were] coming out and saying, 'You know what? My community is deeply anti-Black, and I want to challenge that.'"[17]

Several projects in New York City install "accountability partners," a council of people committed to ensuring the integrity of the project and willing to be in a formal position of reflecting back what they see from their positionality. Three cisgender men, two of them white and one Black, edited the anthology *Letters from Young Activists* in 2005. In recognizing their positionality, they decided to have accountability partners composed mostly of women of color, to raise the awareness and network of the project and recommend contributors who they would be wise to include. In 2009, the Challenging Male Supremacy Project, which conducted nine-session cohorts of men (cis and trans) through topics of desire, violence, and feminist analysis, also incorporated accountability partners, composed mostly of leaders of organizations of queer people of color, trans folks, and cisgender women. The accountability partners reviewed and discussed the Challenging Male Supremacy Project's curriculum and met to provide feedback for the facilitators. "Liberation cannot be experienced through introspection alone or while waiting for others to point out places of oppression.... We must, all of us, openly acknowledge the real norms, desires, biological myths, and practices that fuel racial, sexual, and gender-based hatred. Our collective liberation requires that society, which is a collective body, turn within to face and dissolve the hatred that has claimed our lives," Zenju Earthlyn Manuel encourages us.[18] The facilitators wanted their work of interrogating male supremacy to be accountable to organizations led by people of color and queer folks who they enlisted as accountability partners, and the accountability partners agreed to be in this formal position of providing feedback and making requests of the facilitators. Utilizing the practice of accountability partners builds community, anticipates dissonance and the lack of awareness generated by privilege, and ensures that one's work serves those most affected by systems of oppression.

Resource Generation organizes young people with wealth. The organization holds an annual conference in which there is a ritual of standing in a circle and revealing where one's family's wealth comes from: sales of weapons, lead paint, pharmaceuticals, cotton, railroads. Participants work out their family money story in small groups, then larger groups, and then in front of the entire conference, slowly building their courage and titrating their own exposure to the discomfort of what they share within and beyond their own bodies. The understanding within the organization is that transparency and truthfulness is part of healing. Tessa Hicks Peterson explains, "Those who are assigned dominant roles in terms of power, access, privilege, and reputation obviously benefit directly from their positionality, but they are also negatively affected by having their investments, benefits, and sense of self-worth tied to a hierarchal system in which they succeed at the expense of others."[19]

When Resource Generation members are clear about their wealth history and family history, it allows them perspective on what kind of healing they need personally and where to allocate their family's resources. One white queer member, Karen Pittelman, created a foundation with people of color on the board who decided which organizations her inheritance would support. Resource Generation members discuss reparations, directing giving plans toward healing the oppression and pain created by their family's accumulation of wealth. Their transparency and honesty fuels their practice of healing the harm done to so many people. Scholar and yoga teacher Becky Thompson states, "In the end, there can be no enlightenment without an acknowledgement of the forces that divide us from one another, no inner peace without striving to create peace for everyone."[20]

Callouts can be a useful, temporary tactic to halt harm, a way to demand accountability when other strategies are halted. It can be an effective tactic when someone is not recognizing the harm they've caused, or their power and privilege protect them from accountability—in these cases it can even ignite the transformative process. "Calling people out shuts down listening and escalates the conflict," Black feminist Loretta Ross points out.[21] This can be useful to draw attention to something and strategically elevate tension. As adrienne maree brown advises, "There is absolutely a need for certain call outs—when power is greatly imbalanced and multiple efforts have been made to stop ongoing harm, when someone accused of harm won't participate in community accountability processes, the call out is a way of pulling an emergency brake."[22] This is a tool, and it should be used intentionally and with purpose, rather than universally applied. As often as possible, we must respond in a generative and healing way, rather than with a callout—a way that can lead to growth rather than escalation of conflict.

Calling out can be destructive within organizations, communities, and movements, and not only can hurt the people at the center or involved peripherally but also the surrounding bystanders as well. At the Allied Media Conference in 2017, Black Lives Matter co-founder Alicia Garza said, "Colonization, capitalism, imperialism, white supremacy, heteronormativity, patriarchy—all of these systems function to break the bonds of relationship between us. Our movement must be a different one. One that seeks to forge many different kinds of relationships that reject the systems that tear us apart, rejects the fear and hatred and that rejects power over in favor of power with."[23] Many in our movements and potential participants fear that they will make a mistake and be shunned like others they have witnessed, and so they shut down their creativity, are reluctant to take risks, withdraw, or don't show up to begin with. Isn't that the opposite of what will allow our movements to be big, powerful, successful, and alluring? Isn't that fear of joining counterproductive?

Many instances of callouts within our communities and movements result from blame, shame, reactivity, performances of who is right and who is wrong, and public displays of private conflicts. This idea of callouts is that we will shame one another into being better. We will isolate each other into self-reflection. We will interrupt someone's work in the interest of their growth. But as adrienne maree brown asks us, what is at stake if we move against ourselves? Callouts cause many people to leave social movements, sever impactful collaborations and relationships, and alter individuals' lives significantly. Calling out has halted broader work as we fight among ourselves. Loretta Ross points out, "Most public shaming is horizontal and done by those who believe they have greater integrity or more sophisticated analyses. They become the self-appointed guardians of political purity."[24]

Maisha Z. Johnson suggests, "Addressing harmful behavior is important, but so is understanding that everyone is on a different step of their journey, so we all make mistakes.... You don't have to shame other activists—or yourself—for being imperfect. We can give ourselves and each other room to make mistakes."[25] When confronted by our own mistakes or those of a colleague, we might turn toward the practices laid out in part 1 of this book, remembering each other's basic goodness, forgiving ourselves and each other for being a student of life and making mistakes, and practicing acceptance of the way things are and the way things have been, which in turn makes space for creativity, imagination, and vision of a different way of being.

What does it mean to stay in relationship through those conflicts, rather than giving up on one another? The invitation adrienne maree brown makes is "to see individual acts of harm as symptoms of systemic harm, and to do what we can to dismantle the systems and get as many of us free as possible."[26] Alicia Garza reminds us of the bigger picture of where we are headed: "It won't be easy. We will disappoint each other. Make each other mad. We will hurt each other and we will make mistakes. We will disagree. Building a movement across difference for the sake of our collective transformation is that task of our generation and the generations that we will fight for to succeed us."[27]

These moments of conflict are precisely why our internal spiritual practices matter in social justice work—we can't just do work on policies and practices, building organizations and organizing campaigns. Alicia Garza continues, "No movement has ever been built without people who have disappointed you. That's because movements themselves are the places where people are called to transform in the service of their own liberation and the liberation of others."[28] We must have practices to hold what the outer transformation demands of our hearts. My spiritual practice calls me to act, to speak, to orient toward liberation. And my organizing work demands that I do the inner work to hold the ten thousand joys and the ten thousand sorrows that I encounter along the way so that I can remain present to all of it for the long haul.

Relationship and Fellowship

Through relationship we humanize one another, which is essential to preventing and ceasing the violence and hatred across difference. Kazu Haga reflects in his book *Healing Resistance,* a reflection on Kingian Nonviolence and modern social movements, "Building Beloved Community is not about loving the people who are easy to love. It is about cultivating love for those that are difficult to love. *Those people* over there. The *others.* Those who root for the LA Lakers. The people who voted for *that guy.* The people who work in the very systems that are destroying our communities. The corrupt corporate CEO. The foreign dictator responsible for countless deaths."[29]

Dehumanization is a tool of oppression; humanizing is a tool of liberation. Zenju Earthlyn Manuel says, "It is easier to take land, culture, and language from or commit genocide against a group of people when their identities, their natural appearances, have been distorted into something monstrous."[30] Humanizing anyone deemed as "other" is essential in our path to liberation. This could mean people who wield power over you, or it could be those you consider inferior, misguided, broken, or messy. When we seek to have relationships with those deemed as "something monstrous," we create connection and healing and live into possibility. When there is connection, the dehumanization that Zenju Earthlyn Manuel describes is not possible, for as Desmond Tutu and Mpho Tutu van Furth remind us, "We are created for fellowship. We are created to form the human family, existing together because we were made for one another. We are not made for exclusivity or self-sufficiency but for interdependence. We break this essential law at our own peril. We take care of our world by taking care of each other—it is as simple and difficult as that."[31]

Jesuit priest Gregory Boyle lays out the role that relationship across difference provides in our social change work:

> Our locating ourselves with those who have been endlessly excluded becomes an act of visible protest. For no amount of our screaming at the people in charge to change things can change them. The margins don't get erased by simply insisting that the powers-that-be erase them. The trickle-down theory doesn't really work here. The powers bent on waging war against the poor and the young and the "other" will only be moved to kinship when they observe it. Only when we can see a community where the outcast is valued and appreciated will we abandon the values that seek to exclude.[32]

Angela Davis asks, "Don't we want to be able to imagine the expansion of freedom and justice in the world ... in Turkey, in Palestine, in South Africa, in Germany, in Colombia, in Brazil, in the Philippines, in the US? If this is the case, we will have to do something extraordinary: We will have to go to great lengths. We cannot go on as usual. We cannot pivot the center. We cannot be moderate. We will have to be willing to stand up and say no with our combined spirits, our collective intellects, our many bodies."[33] As we lean into our practice, which declares that change is inevitable, and utilize its timeless tools for adapting and expanding, we fertilize the possibility of so much more than our families and lineages imagined.

What Does Your Heart Break Into?

For many, the very desire to work on specific issues of social concern arises from a personal experience with that same conflict or pain. We must be committed, then, to consciously and consistently reflect on our own healing around this issue, so that, as Hala Khouri says, "we become empowered to act from a place of awareness and compassion rather than an impulsive agenda motivated by our fear and our wounds."[34] Desmond Tutu and Mpho Tutu van Furth suggest, "We must do everything possible to dig the hurt out at the very roots that have bound us to it for so long. And the only way to reach the taproot is with the truth. It has often been said that we are as sick as the secrets we keep. Often the initial harm done to us is compounded by our own shame and silence about what we have suffered.... We are not responsible for what breaks us, but we can be responsible for what puts us back together again."[35]

When we do the work of transforming policies and institutions that have harmed us, if we are not healing on the inside as well we may hurt others along the way, perpetuate harm in our work and relationships, and, perhaps, we ourselves will burn out. When we heal, our work becomes more grounded, strategic, and sustainable. For most of us, in our work we will encounter triggers, for we are directly putting ourselves in relationship with that which harmed us. We need qualities of gentleness and steadiness in order to know that justice begins in our own bodies. Mindfulness and embodiment practices can help, as Becky Thompson describes: "Over time, you alter how you respond to the triggers that revive your experience of trauma. And when you learn how to stay steady in the face of those triggers, you will see the trauma from a different perspective."[36]

Part of healing the trauma of injustice is turning toward the oppression, guilt, shame, or fear that we internalize   the part of ourselves that believes a stigma or stereotype. When we are honest and transparent about who we are, and work toward loving ourselves fully, it helps remove the stigma and connects us to others who have had that experience specifically, or others who have experienced suffering more generally. It magnifies our humanity, allowing trust, connection, and joy. Becky Thompson instructs us, "When we try to hide a secret, we keep ourselves from each other, maybe from the people who we need the most, who will truly understand."[37] To heal, we must work to know who we are and to love ourselves fully, to surround ourselves with people who understand and support us, and to continue to investigate the ways in which we project our fears of rejection or harm on the world; in that embrace, we become more whole. Cuban American Soto Zen priest Hilda Gutiérrez Baldoquín explains, "It is the nature of oppression to obscure the limitless essence, the vastness of who we are—that the nature of our mind is luminous, like a clear pool reflecting a cloudless sky."[38]

Swami Jaya Devi asks, "What do our hearts break into?" Who do we become in the midst of our heartbreak? How might our potency in the world not be in spite of the oppression that we have endured, but because of it? Alice Walker claims, "A writer's heart, a poet's heart, an artist's heart, a musician's heart, is always breaking. It is through that broken window that we see the world; more mysterious, beloved, insane and precious for the sparkling and jagged edges of the smaller enclosure we have escaped."[39]

In my time in this realm of work intersecting social justice and healing, I have witnessed social justice workers turn toward healing and healers turn toward activism. This is essential. We need each other's historical memory, skills, tools, visions, lived experiences, and networks. We are puzzle pieces that fit together, comprising a larger collective puzzle of inner and outer change, which leads to lasting transformation. When we meet each other in the work, rather than wondering where each other has been, we might rather greet each other with gratitude. Oh you, acupuncturist, you're here to march for Black Lives Matter, thank god! Oh dear one, leading an economic justice organization through a challenging campaign, you're going on meditation retreat for the next three months, yes! Oh wow, a meditation retreat center staff traveled to Standing Rock to be in solidarity with indigenous peoples fighting the Dakota Access Pipeline. Thank you, and roll up your sleeves!

We need as many of us as possible to be doing this inner and outer change work to win. How do we encounter each other, work together, grieve our losses, and overcome our disputes in a way that breaks together, rather than falls apart? How do we keep as many of us in the movement and in relationship as possible, on a daily and annual basis? When we work to heal from the trauma of injustice, we claim our place in the world, we pronounce our resilience, and we create space not only for ourselves but also for anyone who has been marginalized or harmed because of who they are. When there is space for each of us, we incite the potential to thrive collectively and individually. I crave to live into that world.

CONCLUSION:
A PATH FROM HERE

I BOTH CHERISH and disdain yoga and dharma. I feel both honored and ashamed when I share that I am a yoga teacher at a social gathering. As long as yoga is present in the United States and practiced around the world, there is much work to do to honor its roots and manifest its true potential for justice. I love the teachings and, as you can see, they have guided my life; they are a deep guidance toward justice in our world.

If I love something, I must be dedicated to its well-being and integrity; yoga and dharma have some reckoning to do in this world, and in the United States in particular. We must be connected and accountable to the history of these practices; we must know their history as it intersects with international political history, colonization, and resistance to and overthrow of colonial forces. We must honor the lands and peoples from whom these practices came, out of our own practice of generosity and accountability. We can evolve the teachings to explicitly bend toward justice, for they are inevitably ever-evolving. We can work to invite more people in and practice equity in the sharing of the teachings, whether teaching postures, breath, or philosophy. Many are already doing this.

I have some suggestions.

I suggest taking up the ethical practices articulated within Buddhism and yoga to truly live into the liberatory potential of the teachings. I suggest evolving yoga teacher certification and accreditation beyond the two-hundred-hour model. And I suggest both listening deeply to critiques of ourselves and our projects and calling each other in when we fall short, make mistakes, or reproduce oppression.

Ethics and Our Future

Both the five precepts of Buddhism and the Yamas of yoga guide me in a daily way. I agree with Sebene Selassie when she says, "At the core of *any* worthwhile wisdom tradition are ethical teachings. Some of us may have received clear principled guidance (spiritual or secular) from our families and communities. But generally, ethics are rarely explored in modern life outside of professional codes and religious communities. Integrity is the foundation for healthy individuals and society; without it, mayhem ensues (this could explain a lot)."[1] The Yamas and the precepts are the cornerstone of "living our practice," a guiding light for the moments of our days when we may be swayed one way or another. The Yamas and the precepts invite us back to our basic goodness and remind us that we are entitled to our actions but not the fruit of our actions, as Krishna states in the Bhagavad Gita—we follow the ethical practices without expectation of what comes next.[2]

I worry about the field of mindfulness in much the same way that mainstream yoga pisses me off, because neither emphasize the ethical practices. Mainstream yoga is generally yoga asana without the other seven limbs of yoga. Mindfulness is one aspect of the Eightfold Path of Buddhism, without the other seven practices. Without the ethical practices of these tried-and-true traditions, we can teach snipers to better aim and focus, which leads them to kill more effectively. We can teach corporate CEOs how to "de-stress" so that they feel less of the impact of their actions on their own body/heart/mind. We can make yoga and mindfulness into multibillion-dollar industries, even though nonstealing, gratitude, and generosity are present in the ethical practices. It is cultural appropriation if we take what is convenient to the status quo and leave behind what challenges the violent and harmful patterns in our society that make money for the powers that be. When we secularize the teachings, whose interest is served? What is not grappled with? Who are we not accountable to? What can we get away with?

In the chapter on yoga and capitalism, I discussed the Yamas, the ethical practices of yoga that compose its first limb. The five precepts of Buddhism are much the same, swapping out Aparigraha for refraining from intoxication.

Simply, the Buddhist precepts are:

1. Don't create harm.

2. Don't take what's not yours.

3. Use your sexuality skillfully.

4. Be truthful and behave with integrity.

5. Steady your body/heart/mind by not using intoxicants.

Caitriona Reed, a trans Zen teacher who founded Manzanita Village, portrays the Buddhist precepts this way:

1. Aware of the violence in the world and of the power of nonviolent resistance, I stand in the presence of the ancestors, the earth, and future generations, and vow to cultivate the compassion that seeks to protect each living being.

2. Aware of the poverty and greed in the world and of the intrinsic abundance of the earth, I stand in the presence of the ancestors, the earth, and future generations, and vow to cultivate the simplicity, gratitude, and generosity that have no limits.

3. Aware of the abuse and lovelessness in the world and of the healing that is made possible when we open to love, I stand in the presence of the ancestors, the earth, and future generations, and vow to cultivate respect for the beauty and the erotic power of our bodies.

4. Aware of the falsehood and deception in the world and of the power of living and speaking the truth, I stand in the presence

of the ancestors, the earth, and future generations, and vow to cultivate the ability to listen, and to practice clarity and integrity in all that I communicate—by my words and my actions.

5. Aware of the contamination and desecration of the world and of my responsibility for life as it manifests through me, I stand in the presence of the ancestors, the earth, and future generations, and vow to cultivate care and right action, and to honor and respect health and well-being for my body, my mind, and the planet.[3]

These inward practices are deeply impactful, shifting how we show up every moment. Whatever we practice grows stronger. When we individually and collectively practice judgment, alienation, shame, and guilt, although these are inevitable and normal human emotions, we limit our freedom. As my friend Jo Kent Katz says, "Guilt, shame, and blame are not liberatory practices." These ethical practices lead us not toward what is "right" or "good," as opposed to wrong or evil, but toward freedom. In practicing the Yamas and the precepts, we dedicate our lives to the dignity, safety, and belonging of each being.

Transcending the Two-Hundred-Hour Training

In my studies with Swami Jaya Devi, and with every teacher who has profoundly impacted my practice or guided my teaching, I have been taught that I am always a student before I am a teacher. However, despite the longevity and expanse of these practices, which demand a lifetime (at least one lifetime!) of study, Yoga Alliance has supported a two-hundred-hour training model, at the end of which a person is certified to teach yoga. I have some suggestions for students, yoga teachers, and power holders such as Yoga Alliance.

If you are a yoga student, I invite you to query your teachers more deeply about their training and skill set. Your body, nervous system, and heart are in the hands of the teacher; do your homework! Pay attention to how yoga is being offered (as weight loss? stress reduction? for connection? for liberation?) and who keeps coming back (do fat people return? older folks? people with injuries? people of color?). Know what to research in the biographies of teachers, such as years of teaching experience, where they were trained and what lineage that studio or ashram practices within, the level of training they have, if they are engaged deeply in self-study or personal growth in some consistent way, whether they teach just one or two classes a week or teach full time (which means more experience over less time), and what diversity of lived experiences and bodies they have worked with.

In an interaction with your teacher, if you have an injury or condition, ask if they have worked with that specific condition, pay attention to your own embodied experience in the class, and be courageous to not do something that the teacher is instructing if it doesn't feel right in your body. Notice if a teacher places value on one manifestation of a given posture over another—do they say "the full expression of a pose" or "a more advanced posture" or do they say "variation" or another word that doesn't connote a hierarchy of body expression? Demand skillfulness of your teachers, and trust your intuition.

These recommendations are practices in paying attention, lovingkindness, and participating in the integrity of yoga. It's not about scrutiny; it's about recognizing that yoga in the US is complicated and messy and taking responsibility for your own participation and presence.

With respect to teaching, we should abandon two-hundred-hour yoga teacher trainings and instead transition yoga teaching to a four-year advanced degree, with full financial aid programs that are authorized for federal loan forgiveness programs. There are a few advanced degree programs around the country like this, such as Loyola Marymount University's yoga studies master's degree program and a PhD program through the Yoga Research Center that began in 2021. Those who are at the helm of yoga and social justice and those with specialized knowledge within the vast realm of yoga should be hired as professors, centering teachers who have been historically marginalized, especially South Asian leaders with ancestral connection to the practice.

As for the teachers already teaching, I'd like to see continuing education requirements such as those required for therapists and other licensed professions, so that existing teachers are keeping up with new information and ever deepening their studies. If it's not required, then many teachers, especially those with greater social capital, financial backing, and privilege in our society, will go on teaching with just the minimal training hours without being transparent to students and clients about that, and sooner or later they will cause great or more subtle harm. There will certainly be exceptions.

For yoga teachers with a dedication to the history of yoga and a commitment to its future, we must commit ourselves to consistent and never-ending study and being honest about our training. We must responsibly turn down some opportunities and have a referral network of other teachers with skills or training we ourselves don't have and give opportunities to skilled teachers not yet in the spotlight, with special attention to those from marginalized communities. We must direct the future of yoga toward integrity, justice, and equity.

Practicing with Critique

In the years that I co-owned Third Root Community Health Center, we faced countless critiques. We put ourselves out there to truly be a community institution in a very diverse community. We were always going to need help to get there—to reflect the community around us and be in alliance with the communities of color that had populated the Flatbush neighborhood of Brooklyn for decades. We faced more critique than the average yoga studio, acupuncture facility, or massage therapy office—we absorbed the critiques that had been waiting in the wings after so many institutions had just not been able to hear them.

Third Root, as is any project, was imperfect. Each of us practicing justice are imperfect. Writer Frances Lee calls for a politic of imperfection and responsibility in her article in *YES!* magazine based on her experience as a queer, trans, Chinese American, middle-class, able-bodied woman:

> *A politics of imperfection asks me to openly acknowledge the ways in which my family and I have benefited and continue to benefit from oppressive systems such as slavery, capitalism, and settler colonialism. A politics of responsibility means that as I am complicit in harmful systems, I also possess full*

agency to do good. This allows me to commit to dismantling these systems and embracing centuries-long legacies of resistance. It means I am accountable in community spaces and do not destroy myself when others call me out on my errors. It means I practice a generosity of spirit and forgiveness towards myself and others. To do all this, I must publicly claim both imperfection and personal responsibility as an activist.[4]

Frances Lee suggests that a politic of imperfection and responsibility commit us further to the work, rather than letting us off the hook. There are systems at play that are larger than any one of us. As my friend En Wong said at a Buddhist Peace Fellowship Block Build Be retreat in 2017, "It's not my fault, but it is my responsibility."

The Buddha said that we would inevitably encounter blame and disrepute, as I discussed in the chapter on equanimity in part 1. Social movement visionary adrienne maree brown invites us to "take each moment of conflict and harm as practice ground for abolition."[5] We are trying to build a more just world, where conflicts and harm can be addressed by the broader community and can potentially bring us into closer relationship. There are countless examples in restorative justice work, where men who killed each other's best friends become friends and allies, where someone who stabbed another helps the victim heal his trigger at the site of the stabbing, where a mother of a slain child adopts his killer. We have this immense capacity in the midst of conflict to do something extraordinary and incredibly loving, holding the larger vision.

Yoga and Buddhist communities in the US often engage critiques as assaults or problems—a problem created by the person doing the critiquing. Critiques are often opportunities to grow. Don't we all want to grow our hearts to be bigger, to know how to love in a way that is fulfilling in a daily way? Wouldn't the growth being called upon ultimately benefit our communities, our projects, our studios, our trainings?

When engaging critique, we must first ground ourselves—often after taking some space from the critique itself. In the heat of the moment, when your nervous system is rattled, that's a terrible time to examine truthfulness. Use some of your practices, call upon your tools, move your body, deepen your breath, connect with what is most important to you.

Then examine: Is this true? From whose perspective is this true? Am I sure? If it's not true, phew! Let it go and go on living your life, doing your work, cultivating your practice with integrity and kindness. Sometimes you may fight off the falsehood, biting back. Other times you may just let it fade, your continued words and action proving it to be untrue or a brief blip on a screen of otherwise-impeccable kindness and integrity.

If it's true, it's a gift, a reflection, a chance to engage in a different way. Something needs to change to accommodate a group of people or an individual you care about, thereby making your practice or your sangha more caring! That's wonderful! Move slowly and thoughtfully, set up systems of accountability to the person who gave you the gift of critique and their community, if appropriate, and offer to compensate them for their labor. Do the growing that is invited, and continue to resource yourself as you do so with your practice, being even more stringent about practice time while under this pressure. Your practice will allow you to show up to this process of healing with dignity, purpose, and presence.

In response to callout culture, many important thinkers have proposed "calling in," done from a place of love, refusing to give up on one another amid mistakes, and collectively living into deep transformation and, ultimately, liberation. Ngọc Loan Trần proposed in 2013, "I picture 'calling in' as a practice of pulling folks back in who have strayed from us. It means extending to ourselves the reality that we will and do fuck up, we stray, and there will always be a chance for us to return. Calling in is a practice of loving each other enough to allow each other to make mistakes, a practice of loving ourselves enough to know that what we're trying to do here is a radical unlearning of everything we have been configured to believe is normal."[6] In that unlearning, we will make mistakes, again and again. In turning toward one another in such moments, when we have the capacity to do so, we begin ceasing to travel the path of blame and shame and instead forge a revolutionary path created out of forgiveness, accountability, and commitment. Loretta Ross describes it thus: "Calling-in is simply a call-out done with love. Some corrections can be made privately. Others will necessarily be public, but done with respect. It is not tone policing, protecting white fragility or covering up abuse.

It helps avoid the weaponization of suffering that prevents constructive healing."[7]

When we receive critique—as we will, as we must if our world is going to grow into something where everyone has what they need and no one has more than they need—we are invited to sit with critique, to feel our feelings, to remain embodied and breathe, and, once the nervous system settles, to investigate: What can grow from the honesty of that moment? From me individually? From a larger group—the studio, the community, the neighborhood, the city? And when we see one another's mistakes and harm, we must pause for a moment, turning inward and asking: How can this conversation about this harm grow our movement and our community? How can it help us love deeper and wider? How can it take us toward greater transformation? "Call-ins are agreements between people who work together to consciously help each other expand their perspectives," says Loretta Ross. "They encourage us to recognize our requirements for growth, to admit our mistakes and to commit to doing better. Calling in cannot minimize harm and trauma already inflicted, but it can get to the root of why the injury occurred, and it can stop it from happening again."[8] Calling in is a practice of repair, of stopping the cycle of harm.

❧

We have what we need, collectively. We each have a piece of what is needed, and, therefore, each of us is needed. We are in a transformative moment predicted by many cultures and wisdom traditions, a movement toward a liberatory world, and we have what we need to break through. We have tools and wisdom practices. We have intuition and we have study. We have analysis and clarity. We have historical memory and the lessons of history. We have knowledge of what to hold on to and what to never again repeat. We have play and joy and celebration and fun and laughter. We have intersectionality and we have interdependence. We have elders and youth. We have privileges that protect and the experience of being targeted that begets ferocity and fearlessness. We have resources garnered through harmful means, and we have models of reparations and reconciliation. We have leaders and followers, teachers and students. We have hearts that love so deeply and broadly, hearts that can forgive the gravest atrocity and transform that moment into accountability, connection, and commitment. We have relationships across all kinds of difference and human variance. We have birth workers and death doulas, visionaries and behind-the-scenes folks. We have ethical practices that keep us from straying from our values for short-term gain. We have models of accountability and repair. We have an understanding of the human nervous system and trauma, and an understanding of celestial bodies and their impact on humanity. We have models of mutuality and collaboration surrounding humanity in our plant, creature, and fungus relatives. We have breath and body practices. We have song, crafts, dance, art, and theater. We have earth, water, fire, air, and spirit and the practices and people that honor and protect them, people who have done so unceasingly for millennia.

One of my gifts is that I am situated in between places. Between binary genders and sexual orientations. Between social justice and healing practices. I pray that we each bring our own unique gifts, that we cherish the gifts others bring as well, and that we protect one another's dignity, belonging, and safety along the way.

Appendix A
Asana Sequences

YOGA ASANA IS not the entirety of yoga, even though it is often represented as such around the world. At the same time, the postures, movement, and embodiment are *essential* to the yogic path. Regardless of one's body—fat or thin, disabled or nondisabled, flexible or stiff—embodiment is an important element. For some of us, to inhabit with a depth of awareness and kindness a body that has been targeted, shamed, and pathologized over decades and generations is a radical and important act of self-love and belonging. Many yogis are drawn to yoga through the doorway of the physical—whether it is therapeutic (due to injuries or conditions) or for a "workout." From the beginning conceptions of this book, I wanted it to contain asana that centers queer and trans yogis, for us to know and see ourselves in images of practitioners. When anyone, especially marginalized communities, can see themselves in the practice, they are welcomed in. Beloved queers, this is for you.

If you're not queer or trans and you are perusing this portion of the book, notice what arises in your practice when you don't necessarily see yourself in these next pages. This is the experience of Black yogis, non-Black yogis of color, disabled yogis, fat yogis, and, yes, queer and trans yogis. We rarely see images of ourselves in practice. Perhaps in following these sequences modeled by these beautiful queer bodies, you will benefit physically and energetically, and your heart will grow wider and wiser.

I love crafting creative sequences for specific energetic purposes. Teaching yoga for a decade in New York City, my asana practice was heavily influenced by dance and choreography. I teach weekly classes with philosophical themes, committed to teaching more than just asana while I'm teaching embodiment.

What follows are three short sequences drawn by queer illustrator Elvis Bakaitis and based on illustrations of my Queer and Trans Yoga students in Brooklyn. Each has a specific energetic purpose that I hope you find useful when the circumstances of your life require these qualities. Please use an abundance of props and adapt as you need to.

Sequence for Grounding

This is a sequence where we draw on the grounding energy of the earth. We remain close to the ground, do a lot of work with the legs, and spend at least five breaths in each posture, allowing ourselves to move slowly.

To begin, step your feet mat-width apart and bend your knees into a squat. If this is hard on your knees, ankles, or feet, sit on a block here. Breathe in this squat, feeling the soles of your feet connecting with the steadiness of the earth.

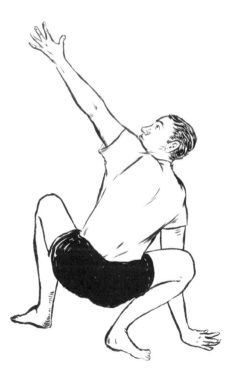

Extend your left arm down and to the left in your twist, and raise the right arm up and back, so that you have a wide wingspan. Take five breaths, return to center, and do the same on the other side.

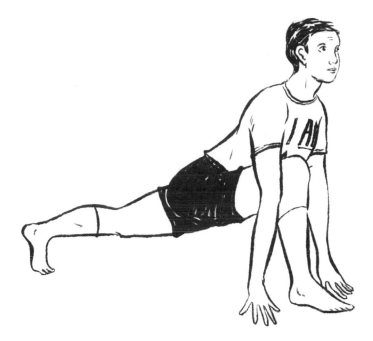

Step your left foot back into a lunge, keeping the back knee up. Extend through the arms and take five slow and steady breaths.

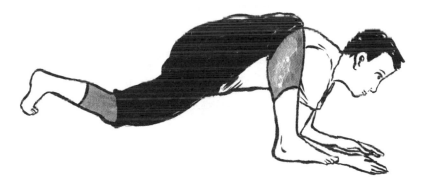

Bring your hands inside your right foot into Lizard Pose, *Utthan Pristhasana*. Lower your left knee. Either stay on your hands or lower your elbows to a block or the ground. Take five breaths here.

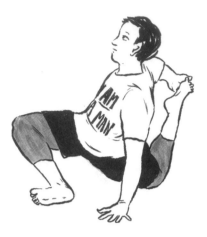

Come to your hands if you were on your elbows, and bring your right hand to your right knee and twist, looking up over your left shoulder. Take five breaths here, and then bend your back knee, raising the foot, and reach back to catch hold of it, stretching the quadriceps and remaining in the twist. If you can't catch your back foot, use a strap or set that foot on a block.

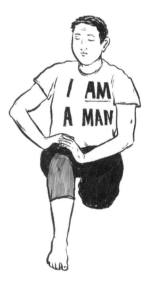

Untwist, step your right foot toward the center of your mat, and bring your hands to your right knee, raising your torso upward and drawing your shoulders back.

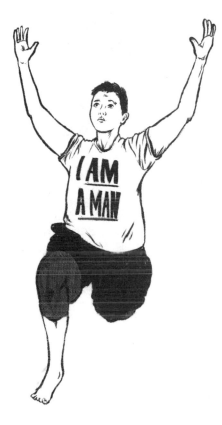

Raise your arms up overhead into *Anjaneyasana*, Crescent Moon Pose, and keep your eyes on the horizon or the ground for further grounding energy. Take five slow breaths here.

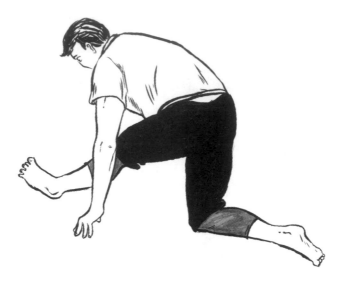

Bring your hands down around your front foot, and lengthen that leg, raising the sole of your foot up off the ground and flexing the left foot. Bow over the left leg, stretching through your hamstrings. Your hands can be on the ground or on blocks if your hamstrings are tight. Take five slow and steady breaths.

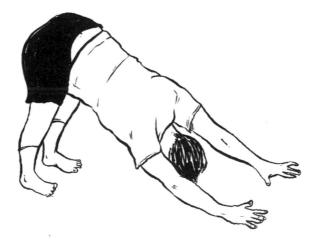

Bend your front knee and step back to Downward-Facing Dog, Adho Mukha Svanasana. Take yourself through a *vinyasa* if you'd like, coming forward to Plank Pose, *Phalakasana*, on an inhale, lowering your knees, chest, and chin on the exhale, raising your chest into Cobra Pose, *Bhujan-gasana,* on the inhale, and returning to Downward-Facing Dog.

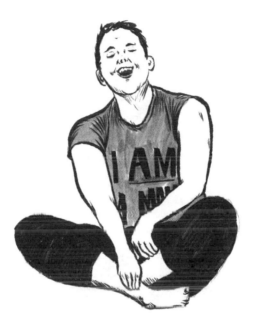

Walk or step your feet forward, lift the heels, and bend the knees deeply, coming into another kind of squat, opening the soles of the feet. Bring your hands to your heart, and twist to the right, hooking your left elbow over your right knee and looking up over your right shoulder. Take three to five breaths here, and then come into a Standing Forward Fold, *Uttanasana,* and continue the sequence on the other side, again taking five breaths in each posture.

Sequence for Fearlessness

In this playful sequence we build energy and heat. It's best to be warmed up before practicing this sequence, so you might take some lunges and Sun Salutations, *Surya Namaskar,* first. This sequence incorporates significant shifts in balance and widening out and folding in, allowing ourselves to take up space, and come in close.

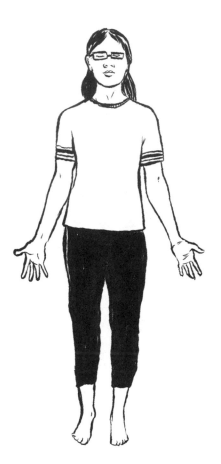

Begin standing in *Tadasana,* Mountain Pose, at the front of your mat.

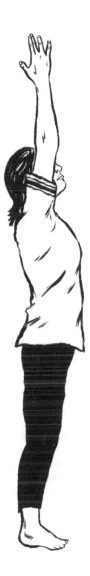

Reach your arms up overhead into *Urdva Hastasana,* Upward Salute.

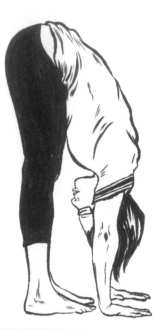

Fold forward over your legs into Uttanasana, Standing Forward Fold.

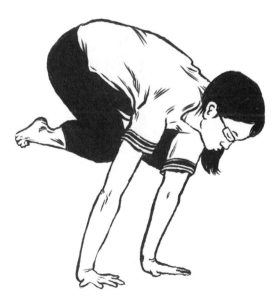

Place your hands on the floor shoulder-width apart, bend your knees halfway into a squat, and begin to transfer your weight to your hands into Crow Pose, *Bakasana.* It can be helpful here to have your feet on a block to help give you lift and/or have a blanket on the floor in front of your face to prevent a face smash. Breathe as deeply as you can as you work to balance on your hands.

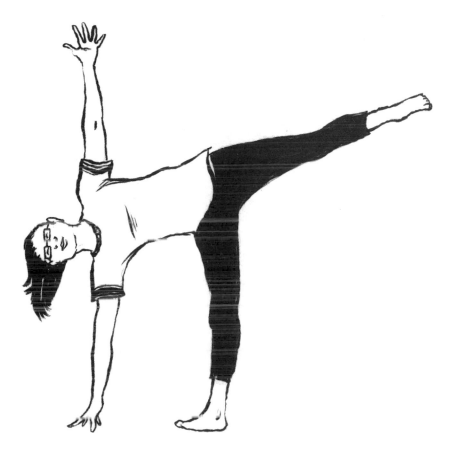

From Bakasana, place your right foot on the ground, open your hips, and extend your left leg back and lift your left hand up into the air, coming into *Ardha Chandrasana,* Half Moon Pose. Extending out from your center, breathe here for five breaths.

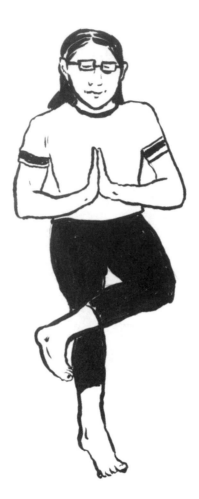

From that balance pose we come into another, Standing Pigeon or Figure Four shape, *Tada Kapotasana*. Bring your left ankle to your right knee, bend your right knee, square your hips, and bring your hands to your heart. Draw your elbows toward your shin, taking breaths through your nose. Take five breaths.

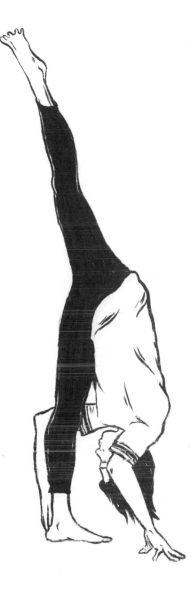

Extend your left leg up into the air, folding forward over your right leg, into Standing Splits, *Urdhva Prasarita Eka Padasana*. You are welcome to have blocks under your hands here, which is especially helpful if the hamstrings are tight. Breathe here for five breaths.

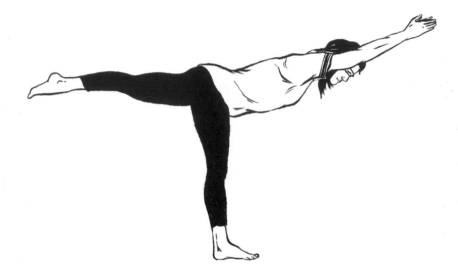

From Standing Splits, we come into Warrior 3, *Virabhadrasana* 3, another balance posture. Start to lower your left leg to parallel with the ground and raise your head, arms, and torso to also be parallel with the ground. Your arms can be outstretched beyond your head, hands can be on your hips, or you can reach the arms out into a *T* position. It can be helpful here to have your hands on blocks at their highest heights for further stability. Extend forward through the top of your head and reach back through your left heel. Slow the breath down, breathing through the nose as best you can, for five breaths.

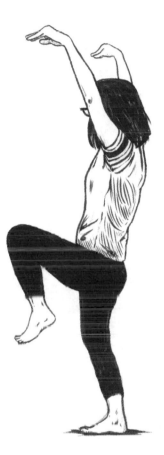

From Warrior 3, tilt your torso upright again, bringing your left knee toward your chest, still standing on your right leg. Bring your arms up into cactus arms, and flick your wrists (how gay, right?!). Start to bend your right knee and fly like a gay graceful crane, this is *Balikikasana,* Crane Pose.

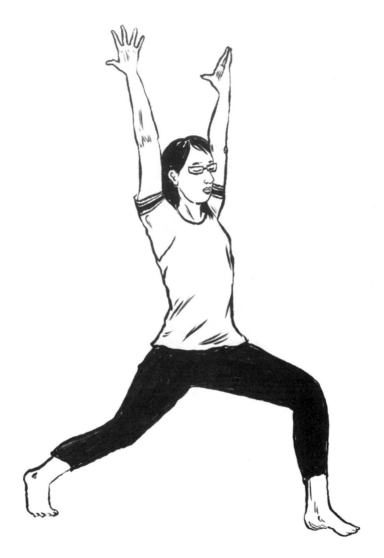

From Balikikasana, step your left foot back three to four feet behind your right foot, landing softly with a bent knee and coming into a high lunge. Lift your arms up into the air and take five breaths.

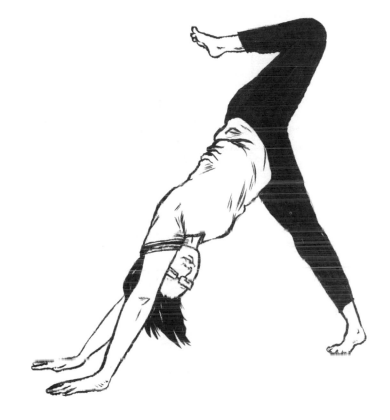

Step back into Downward-Facing Dog, lifting your right leg up into the air, bending the knee, and opening your hips.

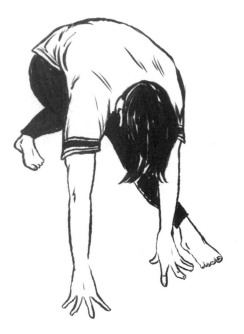

Step your right foot outside your left hand, coming into a Pyramid Pose variation, *Parsvottanasana* variation. Your right pinky toe is outside the pinky of your left hand. Straighten your right leg and press the sole of your foot to the ground. Breathe for five breaths, using blocks if your hamstrings are tight.

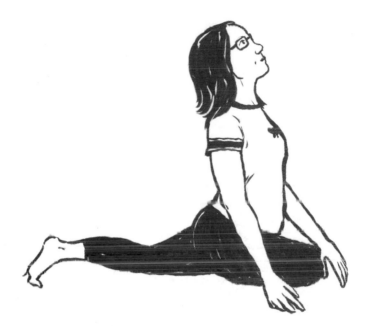

Bend your right knee toward the right wrist, coming into Pigeon Pose, *Eku Puda Rajakapotasana,* and either staying upright or lying down onto the ground. Here we stretch all of the hefty muscles that supported all of the one-legged balance poses.

Repeat the sequence on the left side, trying to move at the same pace, and allow time to rest afterward in Savasana, Relaxation Pose.

Tenderqueer: A Restorative Sequence

This is a gentle sequence to move and care for the body on days when it's difficult to move and care. Perhaps there is something tragic or overwhelming in our world or in your personal life. Move slowly, taking more breaths than usual in each posture, working with deepening the breath moment by moment. Trust the practice to hold you, exactly as you are.

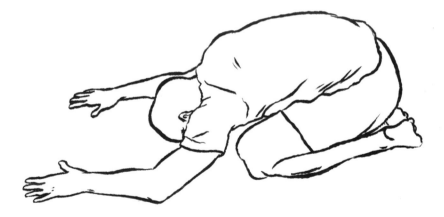

Begin in Child's Pose, *Balasana,* with your knees bent, your forehead on the ground, and your arms stretched out in front of you. Feel the ground holding you, here for you, with whatever you bring to the practice today. Take ten long breaths, breathing through the nose.

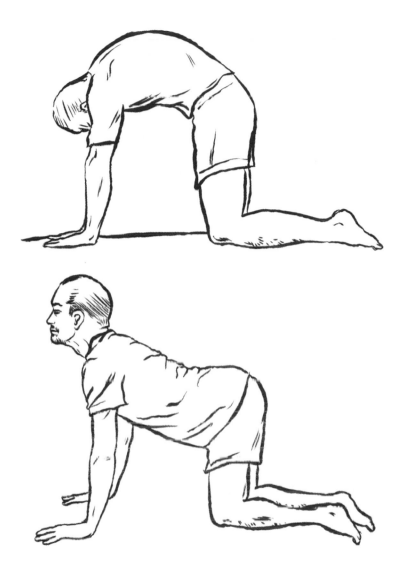

Rise up onto your hands and knees and move your spine into Cat and Cow, *Marjaryasana* and *Bitilasana,* arching the back on an inhale, rounding the back on an exhale. You might place a blanket under your knees to care for your knees if there's any discomfort there. Spend about a minute here moving and breathing.

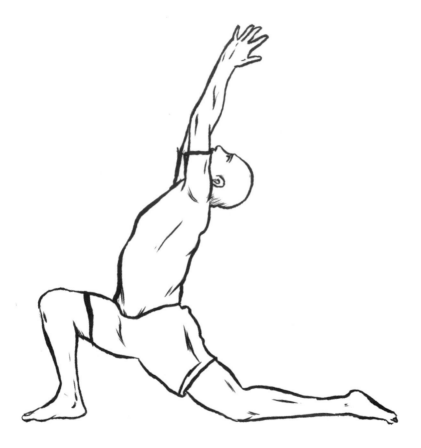

Step your right foot forward between your hands, and reach your arms up overhead, coming into Anjaneyasana. Lift your belly up away from your front thigh, tilt your rib cage back in space, and soften your shoulders as you extend through the elbows.

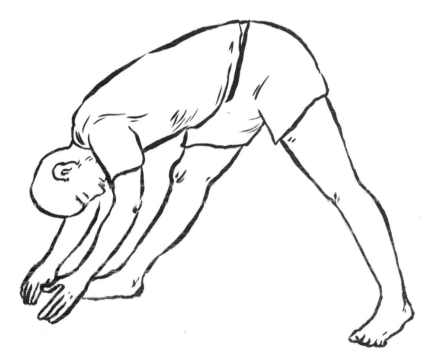

Bring your hands down to the ground or blocks on either side of your right foot, lift your back knee off the ground, and lengthen through your right knee into Pyramid Pose, Parsvottanasana. Breathe seven to ten breaths here.

For five breaths, move between Anjaneyasana and Pyramid Pose, warming up the knee joint.

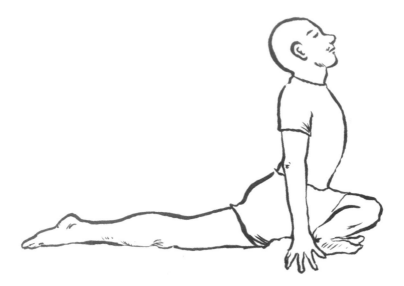

Walk your right foot over to the left, bend your knee, and come into Pigeon Pose. Place a blanket under your right hip, another blanket perhaps on your sacrum, and a block under your forehead, knowing that you are held. Breathe ten long breaths here.

Step back to your hands and knees and repeat Cat and Cow, and then Anjaneyasana, Pyramid, and Pigeon postures on your left side.

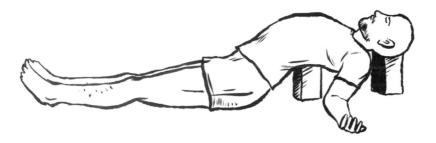

Make your way to a seated position, and set up a block or pillow under your shoulder blades, and another under your head for Supported Fish Pose, *Matsyasana*. Spend three to five minutes here, breathing gently, allowing these props to hold you. Keep bringing awareness back to your breath.

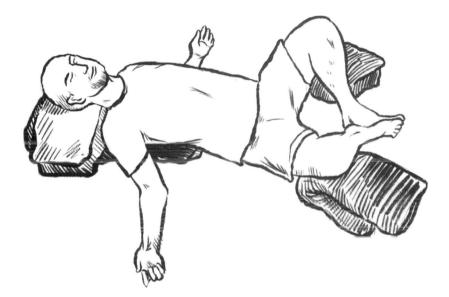

Gently raise yourself up off the props and set up a bolster or two blankets folded into a rectangle about the size of your torso. Sit in front of the bolster or blankets, bring the soles of your feet together into *Baddha Konasana,* Bound Angle Pose, and lie back onto the bolster or blankets. You might take another blanket and lay it over your pelvis here for added grounding and protection. Rest here with your eyes closed or dimmed if you like, in *Supta Baddha Konasana,* Reclining Bound Angle Pose, for three to five minutes, with your arms at your sides and your palms facing up.

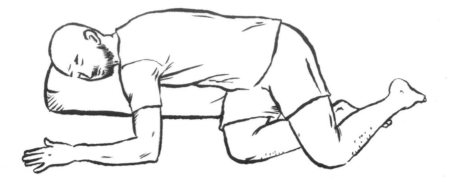

Bring your knees together and roll over to your right side. Turn your torso around so that your belly and chest make contact with the bolster. Turn your head whichever way is most comfortable and breathe in this supported twist for about two minutes. Repeat this on your other side, moving your knees to the other side of the bolster and resting.

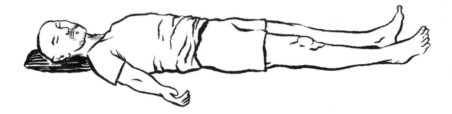

Make your way into Savasana, moving the props you've been using and lying on your back. You might slide a blanket (no higher than one inch) under your head. Allow yourself to rest and be held, staying here for at least five minutes.

Appendix B
Pranayama Practices

BREATH IS WITH us every moment of our life, from the moment we are born to the moment we die. It's a big deal. Most of us don't notice it, and certainly few of us know how to harness its power and influence. *Pranayama* is the fourth limb of the eight limbs of Raja Yoga, preceded by the Yamas, Niyamas, and Asana. Pranayama is the mastery of the life force of the breath. It is said in yogic lore that our life is measured not in years but in breaths; therefore, the longer the breath, the longer one's life. I have worked with children, engineers, nurses, people in recovery, incarcerated folks, college students, athletes, and survivors of sexual trauma. I know without a doubt that breathwork *works*. It's memorable, effective, and powerful.

Prana = energy, vitality/life force

Yama = restriction, observance, control, mastery

Ayama = lack of restriction, release of control over

Putting the words together, therefore, means a mastery of your life force.

Pranayama are breathing exercises developed by ancient yogis and validated by modern scientists. These breathing exercises are used to purify energy channels *(nadis)*, as prana is taken in through the air we breathe. Since the breathing exercises increase the amount of air we take in, they also increase our intake of prana. Prana circulates throughout the body through nadis and energy points that are well understood in Ayurveda and traditional Chinese medicine and it is responsible for all forms of inward reception, from inhalation to eating, drinking, and sensory experiences.

The breath is powerful, and in the yoga tradition, this power is met with great respect, study, and care. Pranayama practices should be approached carefully, ideally with the guidance of a qualified mentor and with self-reflection as to the effects of each technique.

One's state of mind is linked to the flow of breath; therefore, by practicing pranayama you can focus the mind and prepare your attention for the next limbs of the yogic tree: the practices of withdrawal of the senses, concentration, and meditation. Following this progression, it can be useful to practice pranayama at the beginning of a meditation session.

Since the cardiovascular and respiratory systems of the body are connected, when we slow down and deepen the breath the heart has no choice but to slow down. This seems like a basic understanding, one that I learned early in childhood from playing and running. When we take a deep breath, or several over the course of several minutes, the body relaxes. When we speed up and shorten the breath, the body is activated: all systems are in go mode. Sometimes we need to be in go mode. Sometimes we need to chill. Pranayama utilizes this understanding of the body with specific techniques. Some techniques of pranayama are activating, and others are grounding.

Before I present pranayama exercises to work with, let's explore a little bit more the breath's connection with the nervous system, emotions, and the body.

Pranayama, the Nervous System, and Resilience

Many of us have demanding jobs or a role in our family or community where we have to keep showing up, and it can be stressful! The World Health Organization stated that by 2020, depression and anxiety had become the number one disability. In the US, 25 percent of women are taking antidepression medication, antianxiety medication, or both. The CDC has said that sleep disturbances are now at an epidemic level.[1] Breathwork can help.

We live in a stressful world woven with greed, oppression, violence, and environmental degradation. In 2014, as Eric Garner was pinned to the ground in Staten Island, New York, and in 2020, as a police officer knelt on George Floyd's neck in Minneapolis, they each said: "I can't breathe." Each man died soon thereafter, and each killing became one moment (of many) to rally around to protect Black communities from those entrusted to protect. The breaths of individual Black people are disregarded and extinguished. What then does it mean to teach breathwork in a world where many of our siblings and loved ones can't breathe?

Many targeted communities cannot breathe with the systems of oppression and multigenerational trauma bearing down. But what if we learned pranayama techniques as a form of resistance and resilience, knowing that in targeted communities, our breath is not a given? We could internalize and reproduce the threat to our breath, or we could transform it within us so that we can be healthy in an unhealthy world, kind amid cruelty, and our nervous systems could be grounded and balanced despite our communities being under attack. When we are in balance despite the many winds of oppression, injustice, and violence swirling around us, we can make wise (and even visionary!) decisions. If we're caught up in these systems, being blown around without tools such as breathwork, there's a decreased chance that our wisdom will come through in our thoughts, words, and actions. When we act from our wisdom, we can impact the chaos and create a healthier, just world where we can all breathe.

Breathing through the nose calms the nervous system, activating the parasympathetic nervous system (PNS), which is responsible for rest, digestion, and healing. Likewise, exhalation is linked to the PNS: the longer the exhalation, the more activated the PNS. Breathing through the mouth activates the nervous system, turning on the sympathetic nervous system (SNS), which is responsible for fight, flight, freeze, and appease. The inhalation is linked to the SNS—the shorter the inhalation, the more activated the SNS. Breathing through the mouth allows an immediate reception of air and prana, whereas breathing through the nose is more sustainable, as the nostrils filter, warm, and moisten the breath.

Every breath we take, then, is activating and/or grounding the nervous system, automatically and unconsciously. We can learn to work with these patterns to gear ourselves up for a big event or settle ourselves down to rest. For those of us who live in communities targeted by violence, we can learn to be self-regulated through pranayama as a tool of resistance, resilience, and self-preservation.

Stanford Research Institute studied combat vets who returned from Afghanistan with PTSD, teaching them yoga asana and breathwork. Breathwork was the most effective. After three months, their PTSD symptoms were gone, and they remained gone a year later.[2] Every day twenty veterans take their own lives—again, breathwork can be a tool that saves lives. The US Department of Defense is now advocating breathwork and yoga for veterans.[3] Sundar Balasubramanian, a cell biologist, found more nerve growth factor in people who practice pranayama, even for just four to five minutes.[4] Nerve growth factor is a protein needed for neurons to grow. Breathwork can help our nerves grow and connect!

Breath and Emotion

There is a connection between breath and emotion. You cannot have an emotion in your body longer than seven seconds unless you fuel it. When we encounter something that's difficult to feel, we try to suppress it, and we stop breathing. As Nikki Myers says, "the issues are in our tissues."

For every emotion, there is a corresponding breath pattern. Thus, our breath can tell us a lot about how we are doing—grounded, content, excited, anxious—even if we are not able to locate those emotions specifically. We are often most aware of our breath during a crisis, or a panic attack. When we feel contentment or satisfaction, we often take a big breath in and let out a satisfying sigh. We can consciously create this effect in the body, taking advantage of the body's natural patterns, which is the practice of pranayama.

If you suppress grief, and layer it with further grief events, it comes out as anxiety. The energy of that grief cannot be destroyed; it's going to show up somewhere. When people who have high levels of anxiety learn breathing exercises, they often begin to weep. All of us have been taught to suppress grief, especially folks socialized as men. Collectively, we don't know how to grieve—often friends scatter or avoid you; they don't know what to do. And that creates further isolation.

In years of practice and study, I have learned that it is biologically impossible to have an anxiety or panic attack when you are breathing slowly, fully, and steadily. This is important because we spend so much time and money on the symptoms (anxiety and depression) instead of the remedy and prevention (breathwork is both!). What would happen if our children all learned breathing techniques in school? What would happen if our meetings began with breath exercises? What if subway conductors or radio talk show hosts reminded us all to breathe at rush hour?

In a classroom with children, I can energize the room after just thirty seconds of activating breathwork or relax the room in the same time period with grounding breaths—and I do feel like a magician in teaching pranayama to children. Practitioners feel better after even a short practice because they are breathing well, which in turn integrates their emotions and regulates their nervous systems.

Connecting Asana and Pranayama

Moving through the asanas with breath awareness is key to creating a flowing practice and focused attention. This is one thing that differentiates asana from other physical movement practices. "Moving with an awareness of breathing" does not mean you have to (or should) always practice asana with a specific pranayama technique.

When we inhale, we arch the back a little. When we exhale, we round the back a little. There is this constant relationship between the movement of the spine and our breath, which we can draw and expand upon in asana practice.

Basic guidelines for moving with the breath:

- Inhale as you expand the lungs and torso; exhale as you contract the lungs and torso

- Inhale as you extend your arms, legs, or head away from the torso; exhale as you draw them toward the body

- Use *Ujjayi* Pranayama as you practice static poses (see below for instructions for this breath)

- Notice when you hold the breath or when the breath is heavy or labored; this may be an invitation to back off, to do less, to be gentle

The Diaphragm

The diaphragm is a parachute-shaped muscle that connects all along the inside of the torso, with the heart sitting above it and the abdominal organs beneath it. It is this muscle that separates the chest cavity from the abdominal cavity. It acts as a bellows, creating pressure changes in the lungs, drawing oxygen into the lungs, or pushing carbon dioxide out. Even though it feels like we draw air in and push it out, it is actually the pressure change that determines this! Yoga postures and pranayama may have a toning effect on the internal organs. At rest, the diaphragm forms a dome-like shape. When engaged, it expands out and down, making more room for the lungs to expand with breath. This movement creates a shape change for the abdominal organs, so it may appear like we are breathing into our belly. As we exhale, the diaphragm releases and returns to its domed shape. This is the single most important muscle aiding respiration.

Posture

Sitting upright with the spine aligned, the chest open, and the head level allows the lungs to be their most expansive and facilitates the flow of prana. In a slouched posture it is harder to get in a deeper breath, depriving yourself of this prana and literally producing depressed emotions because of the depressed posture. Sometimes if you are unable to draw in a deeper breath it's useful to place a hand on the belly or rib cage or lie down to feel the breath in a deeper way.

Some lineages of yoga practice pranayama in asana, standing or lying belly down or belly up. In other yoga lineages students are taught pranayama practices in a propped, reclined position for quite some time before "graduating" to seated focused breathing. If you are engaging pranayama exercises while seated, it's useful to be seated up on something, to enhance the uprightness of the torso and access the full capacity of the lungs.

Kumbhaka: Breath Retention

Kumbha means a pot—full or empty. *Kumbhaka* is the art of retaining the breath in a state of suspense. The goal of kumbhaka is to free the *chitta* (awareness) from passion and hatred, greed and lust, pride and envy. Chitta and prana become one in kumbhaka. A kumbhaka aids *pratyahara,* the withdrawal of the senses that is the fifth limb of yoga and leads toward meditative practices.

Sahita Kumbhaka is holding the breath in or holding the breath out, intentionally. *Kevala Kumbhaka* is when a practitioner holds the breath out, either intentionally or unintentionally.

B. K. S. Iyengar notes that if you hold a kumbhaka beyond your capacity, the nervous system may be damaged. So watch for warning signs of the sympathetic nervous system getting turned on. If the rhythm of the inhale or exhale is impeded by the kumbhaka, lessen the retention. Advanced practitioners can engage the *bandhas* (energy locks located at the throat, abdomen, and pelvic floor) while holding kumbhakas; beginners will not use the bandhas.

Contraindications: heart or chest problems; with open eyes, kumbhaka that irritates the eyes or turns the face red.

Grounding Pranayama Practices

Breath of Hesitation

Just focusing our attention on the breath enhances our entire awareness. The Breath of Hesitation is a simple practice of taking a breath before responding to something. This isn't necessarily categorized as a pranayama, but it can provide a profound shift, allowing you to respond from a more grounded nervous system rather than react from an activated nervous system. Just the space of one or two deep breaths can bring you back to your values and commitments in this life, reminding you of what is important and putting any interaction into perspective. The Breath of Hesitation can change what you feel, the tone you speak with, and what you choose to say, allowing it to come from a deeper, wiser place.

In the middle of conversation, pause and take a deep breath, and see what happens.

Ujjayi Pranayama

Ujjayi is a common yoga breath, sometimes called "ocean-sounding breath" or translated from Sanskrit as "victoriously uprising," which refers to the rising up of prana within the body through breathing in this manner. Ujjayi helps relieve the body of excess phlegm, warms the breath so the lungs can better absorb it, and strengthens the nervous system.

TECHNIQUE

Sit in a comfortable pose or use this breath through every asana. Inhale through the nose, drawing the sound of the breath from the base of the throat and engaging the glottal muscle. It should make a hissing sound, an *H* sound, or a "Darth Vader" sound. Exhale through the nose with the same sound at the base of the throat. To learn to engage the glottal muscle to make the sound, you might try breathing as if you are fogging a piece of glass.

Dirgha Pranayama

This breath is called the Diaphragmatic Breath or complete breath, because it utilizes the capacity of the lungs. This breath can also illuminate if you happen to be a "reverse breather"—someone whose torso contracts with the inhale and expands with the exhale. This breath calms the mind, allows a complete exchange of air in the lungs, releases tension in the chest and abdomen, and provides a gentle massage to abdominal organs, improving digestion.

TECHNIQUE

Sit in Easy Pose *(Sukhasana)* or Hero's Pose *(Virasana)* and relax your abdomen. Place your palms on your belly and breathe into your lower lungs, feeling your diaphragm drop and your belly expand into your palms. Shift your palms onto your rib cage and breathe into the rib cage, feeling it expand into your sides. Place your fingertips onto the top of your chest, below the collar bones, and breathe into your upper chest, feeling your hands lifting. Exhale completely, gently contracting the abdomen and squeezing out residual air. Repeat this breath pattern several times at the beginning of the class to ground, or throughout asana practice.

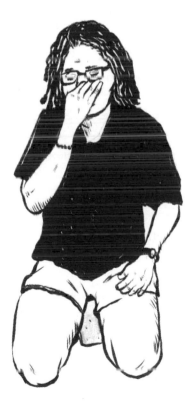

Nadi Shodhana Pranayama

Sometimes called Alternate Nostril Breath, this breath practice helps balance the flow of prana in the body. Typically we breathe dominantly through one nostril for approximately two hours, then we switch sides. This is our natural rhythm! *Nadi Shodhana* purifies the nerve channels, the nadis, and prepares the body for more advanced pranayama.

This breath is also said to balance out the dualities in our bodies—the hot and cold, the quick and slow, the clear and obscure, the rough and smooth, the heavy and light. Any of these qualities out of balance can create illness or unease; therefore, this is a profoundly balancing breath.

TECHNIQUE

Sit in Easy Pose or Hero's Pose. Bring the right hand into Vishnu Mudra, curling the first two fingers into the center of the palm and keeping the thumb and the last two fingers extended. Close the right nostril with the thumb and inhale through the left nostril. Switch your hand, covering the left nostril with the smaller two fingers, and exhale. Inhale through the left nostril, switch your hand to again cover the right nostril with the thumb, and exhale. Continue for three to eleven minutes.

Anuloma Viloma Pranayama

Similar to Nadi Shodhana, this breath practice involves breathing in through one nostril and out through the other and balances dualities. However, the difference is that this is a ratio breath and includes a kumbhaka, or retention, and therefore is a more advanced pranayama practice. The ratio used here is 1 (inhale): 4 (kumbhaka): 2 (exhale).

TECHNIQUE

Begin working with a 3:12:6 ratio. Bring the right hand into Vishnu Mudra, curling the first two fingers into the center of the palm and keeping the thumb and the last two fingers extended. Close the right nostril with the thumb and inhale through your left nostril for three counts. Hold the breath in for twelve counts. Switch your hand, covering the left nostril with the smaller two fingers, and exhale for six counts. Inhale through the left nostril, switch your hand to again cover the right nostril with the thumb, and exhale. Continue for several minutes. You are welcome to increase or decrease the ratio, maintaining an awareness of any tension created from higher counts, and decreasing the ratio if noticed.

Sitali Pranayama

Sitali is a cooling moon breath, strengthening *apana,* or down and outward moving energy, calming the nervous system, cooling the body temperature, and enhancing the eliminative force of the body. It aids digestion, urination, impotence, menstruation, and exhalation. It enhances a slow, steady exhale which stimulates the parasympathetic nervous system. Note that some tongues do not curl, due to genetics—so these folks should breathe in over a flat tongue. This may feel silly, and it may look silly! Perhaps you can try it on regardless, practicing embracing the silly in life.

TECHNIQUE

Sit comfortably in Easy Pose or in a squat. Curl the tongue like a straw and stick the tongue a little way out of the mouth. Inhale through the curled tongue; exhale through the nose. Continue for three to eleven minutes.

Ganga Pranayama

In India, the Ganges River is considered to be the Mother of India, with all of her life-giving bounty. The English name is the River Breath, and following the Standing Rock Water Protectors campaign, to me it honors water everywhere. Practicing the River Breath, imagine yourself drenched in a river of life, of love, in the flow of being. Here we are working with a kumbhaka, which is considered an advanced breath practice. It is important not to struggle with this breath, as it is a ratio breath. Beginners may start at 3:12:6:3; more advanced practitioners may work toward 6:24:12:6.

There are two places to watch the River Breath—the exhalation and the retention of the breath out. Often, after holding the breath in, you may expel the breath too quickly than the full count; try to spread out the exhalation to last for the full count or adjust the ratio to be more workable. Similarly, when holding the breath out, if it feels too long, adjust the ratio.

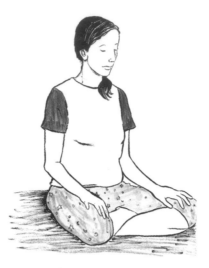

TECHNIQUE

Sit comfortably in Easy Pose. Picture yourself by a sacred river. Choose your ratio. For example, if you are working with a 4:16:8:4 ratio, inhale for a count of four, hold the breath in for sixteen counts, exhale for eight counts, and hold the breath out for four counts. Continue for three to eleven minutes or ten to forty breath cycles.

Activating Pranayama Practices

Bhastrika Pranayama

Bhastrika is also called Bellows Breath because it uses the body like a bellows, powerfully pumping air in and out of the lungs. Bhastrika oxygenates the body and clears the circulatory system, nervous system, and nadis. It helps clear the mind and generate energy, or *kundalini*.

TECHNIQUE

Inhale through the nose, raising the arms overhead and expanding the lungs, rib cage, belly, and abdomen. Exhale powerfully through the mouth, contracting the diaphragm and drawing the arms down at the sides, with the hands clenched in fists. Continue with powerful, rapid inhalations and exhalations. To end, inhale and retain the breath for a few seconds, circulating energy and prana throughout the body; exhale and relax.

Kapalabhati Pranayama

Kapalabhati is also called Breath of Fire. This breath stimulates the third chakra, regulating our health and vitality. It is also a cleansing breath that boosts the immune system, cleanses the blood, and energetically clears what is not needed, thereby increasing our health and vibrancy.

TECHNIQUE

Sit in Easy Pose. Breath of Fire is a rapid, short, powerful breath, focusing on the exhale. To begin, inhale one-third of a breath and exhale forcefully as you pull the navel toward the spine. Repeat. Begin slowly. Speed and coordination come with balance, building toward one breath per second. After the exhale, as you release the belly, breath comes back in, but it won't feel like an inhalation necessarily. To learn this movement of the abdomen, notice the engagement of the belly when you blow out a candle; to find the movement of kapalabhati, engage in the same way but breathe out through the nose.

Kapalabhati also increases core strength and prepares the abdominal muscles for *agni sara,* a hatha yoga practice where a practitioner "stirs" or churns the abdomen, either side to side or in a circle.

Three-Part Standing Breath, Breath of Joy

This breath is a dynamic standing breath to open the chest and lungs and warm the entire body. It is a great way to release frustrations, let go, and reenergize. With beginners it should be practiced more slowly; with regular yogis it can be flamboyant and wild.

TECHNIQUE

Stand with the feet hip-width apart. You will inhale in three parts through the nose, and exhale through the mouth in one breath with sound.

Inhale one-third of a breath as you extend your arms in front of you, palms facing down. Inhale another third of the breath as you extend your arms out wide at shoulder level. Inhale another third of the breath as you bring your arms back to center and then above you. Exhale out your mouth, and swing the arms and torso down, bending the knees and exhaling completely.

Notes

Acceptance and Letting Go

1 Shanesha Brooks-Tatum, "Subversive Self Care: Centering Black Women's Wellness," *The Feminist Wire*, November 9, 2012, https://thefeministwire .com/2012/11/subversive-self-care-centering-black-womens-wellness.

2 Audre Lorde, *A Burst of Light: And Other Essays* (Ithaca, NY: Firebrand Books, 1988), 130.

3 Combahee River Collective, "A Black Feminist Statement" (1977), in *This Bridge Called My Back: Writings by Radical Women of Color*, 4th ed. (Albany: State University of New York Press, 2015).

4 Jack Kornfield, *The Book of Lovingkindness, Forgiveness, and Peace* (New York: Bantam Dell, 2008), 22.

Anger and Sustainability

1 Lama Rod Owens, *Love and Rage: The Path of Liberation through Anger* (Berkeley, CA: North Atlantic Books, 2020).

2 Christopher Ingraham, "Three Quarters of Whites Don't Have Any Non-white Friends," *Washington Post*, August 25, 2014, www.washingtonpost.com /news/wonk/wp/2014/08/25/three quarters-of-whites-dont-have-any-non -white-friends; Seth Adam and Matt Goodman, "Number of Americans Who Report Knowing a Transgender Person Doubles in Seven Years, According to New GLAAD Survey," GLAAD, September 17, 2015, www .glaad.org/releases/number-americans-who-report-knowing -transgender-person-doubles-seven-years-according-new.

3 Domestic workers and farm workers are excluded from federal labor protections such as minimum wage, safety laws, health laws, and the right to a union. Domestic worker organizations have been passing Domestic Workers' Bills of Rights state by state. National Domestic Workers Alliance, "New York," accessed May 25, 2021, www .domesticworkers.org/bill-of-rights/new-york.

Compassion: The Violence Stops with Me

1 Kazu Haga, *Healing Resistance: A Radically Different Response to Harm* (Berkeley, CA: Parallax Press, 2020), 107.
2 Yoga Journal and Yoga Alliance, *The 2016 Yoga in America Survey,* January 2016, www.yogaalliance.org/Portals/0/2016%20Yoga%20in %20America%20Study%20RESULTS.pdf.
3 Dhammapada 1:5 (trans. Gil Fronsdal).
4 Kelly McGonigal, *The Upside of Stress: Why Stress Is Good for You (and How to Get Good at It)* (London: Vermilion, 2015), 154–8.
5 "Stronger," track 12 on Emmanuel Jal, *Warchild,* Sonic360, 2008.

Forgiveness: Releasing the Burden

1 Naomi Shihab Nye, "Kindness," in *Words under the Words: Selected Poems* (Portland, OR: The Eighth Mountain Press, 1994), 42.
2 Jack Kornfield, "The Ancient Heart of Forgiveness," *Greater Good Magazine*, August 23, 2011, https://greatergood.berkeley.edu/article/item/ the_ancient_heart_of_forgiveness.
3 Fania Davis and Sarah van Gelder, "Can America Heal Its Racial Wounds? We Asked Desmond Tutu and His Daughter," *YES!,* May 29, 2015, www.yesmagazine.org/issue/make-right/2015/05/29/can-america-heal -after-ferguson-we-asked-desmond-tutu-and-his-daughter.
4 Susan Verde, *I Am Human: A Book of Empathy* (New York: Abrams Books, 2018), 11.
5 Tamara E. Holmes, "Toward a Cure: Cities Declare Racism a Public Health Crisis," *YES!,* August 26, 2020, www.yesmagazine.org /issue/black-lives/2020/08/26/racism-public-health-crisis.
6 Hyeain Lee et al., "Impact of Obesity on Employment and Wages among Young Adults: Observational Study with Panel Data," *International Journal of Environmental Research and Public Health* 16, no. 1 (January 2019), https://doi.org/10.3390/ijerph16010139.

7   "Health Coverage of Immigrants," Kaiser Family Foundation, March 18, 2020, www.kff.org/racial-equity-and-health-policy/fact-sheet/health -coverage-of-immigrants/.

8   Miles Schneiderman, "The Page That Counts." *YES!,* August 26, 2020, www .yesmagazine.org/issue/black-lives/2020/08/26/the-page-that-counts-6.

9   "Disability Resources: Statistics," US Department of Labor, accessed September 29, 2020, www.dol.gov/general/topic/disability/statistics.

10   Rhonda Magee, *The Inner Work of Racial Justice: Healing Ourselves and Transforming Our Communities through Mindfulness* (New York: Tarcher Parigee, 2019), 82.

11   Magee, 79.

12   Ruth King, *Mindful of Race: Transforming Racism from the Inside Out* (Louisville, CO: Sounds True, 2018), 42.

13   Jardana Peacock, *Practice Showing Up: A Guidebook for White People Work- ing for Racial Justice* (self-pub., 2016), 11.

14   Martin Luther King Jr., "A Christmas Sermon on Peace," in *The Trumpet of Conscience* (Boston: Beacon Press, 1967), 76–77.

A Tussle with Equanimity

1   Tara Brach, *Radical Acceptance: Embracing Your Life with the Heart of a Buddha* (New York: Bantam Books, 2004), 21.

2   Shunryu Suzuki in David Chadwick, *To Shine One Corner of the World: Moments with Shunryu Suzuki* (New York: Broadway Books, 2001), 3.

3   Brach, 133.

4   R. Buckminster Fuller in Daniel Quinn, *Beyond Civilization: Humanity's Next Adventure* (New York: Crown Publishing Group, 2000), 137.

5   Seane Corn, "Nikki Myers: Yoga Therapy for Recovering Addicts," *Yoga Journal,* September 3, 2015, www.yogajournal.com/teach/nikki-myers -yoga-therapy-recovering-addicts/.

6   Sandy E. James et al., *The Report of the 2015 U.S. Transgender Survey* (Wash- ington, DC: National Center for Transgender Equality, December 2016), www .ustranssurvey.org/reports; "The 1 in 6 Statistic," 1in6, accessed May 10, 2021, https://1in6.org/get-information/the-1-in-6-statistic/; "Statistics," The Center for Family Justice, accessed May 15, 2021, https://centerforfamilyjustice.org /community-education/statistics/; "Where We Stand: Racism and Rape," National Alliance to End Sexual Violence, accessed May 15, 2021, https:// endsexualviolence.org/where_we_stand/racism-and-rape/.

7 "Amita Swadhin," Just Beginnings Collaborative, accessed February 7, 2021, http://justbeginnings.org/swadhin.

8 James Baldwin, "As Much Truth As One Can Bear," *New York Times,* January 14, 1962, www.nytimes.com/1962/01/14/archives/as-much-truth-as-one-can-bear-to-speak-out-about-the-world-as-it-is.html.

We Are Fabulous: An Invitation into Joy

1 Thich Naht Hahn, *The Miracle of Mindfulness: An Introduction to the Practice of Meditation* (Boston: Beacon Press, 1999), 32.

2 Mary Oliver, "The Summer Day," in *House of Light* (Boston: Beacon Press, 1990), 60.

3 Lucille Clifton, "Won't You Celebrate with Me," in *Book of Light* (Port Townsend, WA: Copper Canyon Press, 1993), 25.

4 Jalal al-Din Rumi, "Let the Beauty We Love Be What We Do," in *Rumi: The Book of Love: Poems of Ecstasy and Longing*, trans. Coleman Barks (San Francisco: HarperOne, 2005), 31.

5 "Purim Season Is Here!," Jews for Racial and Economic Justice, January 8, 2017, www.jfrej.org/news/2017/01/purim-season-is-here.

6 Yolo Akili, *Dear Universe: Letters of Affirmation and Empowerment for All of Us* (New York: Micheal Todd Books, 2013), 11.

7 Assata Shakur, "To My People by Assata Shakur (Written While in Prison)," July 4, 1973, http://assatashakur.org/mypeople.htm.

8 Dhammapada 1:1 (trans. Gil Fronsdal).

9 McGonigal, *The Upside of Stress,* 49.

10 Edwidge Danticat, *Breath, Eyes, Memory* (New York: Vintage, 1994), 15.

11 Maha Ghosananda, *Step by Step* (Berkeley, CA: Parallax, 1992).

12 Melody Beattie, *The Language of Letting Go: Daily Meditations on Codependency* (Center City, MN: Hazelden Publishing, 1990), 218.

13 Robin Wall Kimmerer, *Braiding Sweetgrass: Indigenous Wisdom, Scientific Knowledge, and the Teachings of Plants* (Minneapolis: Milkweed Editions, 2013), 327.

14 Maya Angelou, *Celebrations: Rituals of Peace and Prayer* (New York: Random House, 2006), 32.

15 Kimmerer, *Braiding Sweetgrass,* 381.

Loving Ourselves Whole

1 Tim McKee, "The Geography of Sorrow: Francis Weller on Navigating Our Losses," *The Sun,* October 2015, www.thesunmagazine.org/issues/478/the-geography-of-sorrow.

2   Eric Kolvig, "What Matters," October 15, 2015, in *Dharma Seed,* podcast, MP3 audio, 45:53, https://dharmaseed.org/talks/30848.

3   Pat Parker, "For the White Person Who Wants to Know How to Be My Friend," *Callaloo* 23, no. 1 (2000): 73.

4   Sharon Salzberg, *Lovingkindness: The Revolutionary Art of Happiness* (Boston: Shambhala Publications, 1995), 32.

5   Steve Biko, *I Write What I Like: Selected Writings by Steve Biko* (Chicago: University of Chicago Press, 2002), 92.

6   James Baldwin, "They Can't Turn Back," *Mademoiselle,* August 1960.

7   Margaret Cho, *Notorious C.H.O.,* directed by Lorene Machado (New York: Wellspring Media, 2002).

8   Audre Lorde, "A Litany for Survival," in *The Black Unicorn: Poems* (New York: W.W. Norton, 1978), 31.

9   Laverne Cox, "On May 29, 2014, the issue of time magazine which proclaimed the 'Transgender Tipping Point' was revealed with me on the cover," Tumblr, June 2, 2015, http://lavernecox.tumblr.com /post/120503412651/on-may-29-2014-the-issue-of-timemagazine.

10   Salzberg, *Lovingkindness,* 33.

Not Living Our Yoga, Just Selling It: Yoga and Capitalism

1   Carolyn Gregoire, "How Yoga Became a $27 Billion Industry—and Reinvented American Spirituality," *Huffington Post,* December 16, 2013, www.huffpost.com/entry/how-the-yoga-industry-los_n_4441767.

2   Kim Kelly, "What 'Capitalism' Is and How It Affects People," *Teen Vogue,* August 25, 2020, www.teenvogue.com/story/what-capitalism-is.

3   adrienne maree brown, "Capitalism IS a Conspiracy," adrienne maree brown (blog), April 16, 2020, http://adriennemareebrown.net/2020/04/16 /capitalism-is-a-conspiracy.

4   Ned Resnikoff, "Yoga Teachers: Overstretched and Underpaid," MSNBC, July 7, 2014, www.msnbc.com/msnbc/yoga-teachers-overstretched-and -underpaid-msna362746.

5   Resnikoff, "Yoga Teachers."

6   David Korten, "Maybe the Gig Economy Doesn't Have to Mean Oppressed Workers," *YES!,* August 24, 2016, www.yesmagazine .org/economy/2016/08/24/maybe-the-gig-economy-doesnt-have -to-mean-oppressed-workers.

7   Crosby Burns, "The Gay and Transgender Wage Gap," Center for American Progress, April 16, 2012, www.americanprogress.org/issues/lgbtq -rights/news/2012/04/16/11494/the-gay-and-transgender-wage-gap.

8   Tasha Eichenseher, "Is 200 Hours Enough to Teach Yoga?," *Yoga Journal,*
    October 12, 2016, www.yogajournal.com/teach/200-hours-enough
    -teach-yoga.

9   Eichenseher.

10 Jocasta Shakespeare, "Bend it like Bikram," *Guardian,* June 11, 2006,
    www.theguardian.com/lifeandstyle/2006/jun/11/healthandwellbeing
    .features1.

11 Vanessa Grigoriadis, "Karma Crash," *New York,* April 13, 2012, https://
    nymag.com/news/features/john-friend-yoga-2012-4.

12 Alexandra Jacobs, "First Lady of Yoga," *New York Times,* April 5, 2013,
    www.nytimes.com/2013/04/07/fashion/colleen-saidman-yee-the-first
    -lady-of-yoga.html.

13 Resnikoff, "Yoga Teachers."

14 Bethany McLean, "Whose Yoga Is It, Anyways?," *Vanity Fair,* April 2012,
    https://archive.vanityfair.com/article/2012/4/whose-yoga-is-it-anyway.

15 Adam Carney, "Yoga Teachers: How to Maximize Your Profits from Yoga
    Retreats," Book Yoga Teacher Training blog, March 28, 2018, www
    .bookyogateachertraining.com/news/maximize-your-profits-yoga-retreat.

16 Travel.Earth, "Does Voluntourism Do More Harm Than Good?," Medium,
    June 10, 2019, https://medium.com/responsible-travel/does-voluntourism
    -do-more-harm-than-good-db9d0c9aedfe.

17 "COVID-19 Relief Fund 2020 Impact Report," Reclamation Ventures
    Fund, last modified August 16, 2020, https://fund.reclamationventures.co
    /impact.

Cultural Appropriation and Yoga

1   Maisha Z. Johnson, "What's Wrong with Cultural Appropriation? These
    9 Answers Reveal Its Harm," Everyday Feminism, June 14, 2015, https://
    everydayfeminism.com/2015/06/cultural-appropriation-wrong.

2   Olufunmilayo Arewa, "Cultural Appropriation: When 'Borrowing'
    Becomes Exploitation," *Huffington Post,* December 6, 2017, www.huffpost
    .com/entry/cultural-appropriation-wh_b_10585184.

3   Susanna Barkataki, "How to Decolonize Your Yoga Practice," Susanna
    Barkataki (blog), September 25, 2015, www.susannabarkataki.com/post
    /how-to-decolonize-your-yoga-practice .

4   Sheena Sood, "Cultivating a Yogic Theology of Collective Healing: A
    Yogini's Journey Disrupting White Supremacy, Hindu Fundamentalism,
    and Casteism," *Race and Yoga* 3, no. 1 (2018): 18.

5 Barkataki, "How to Decolonize Your Yoga Practice."

6 Tobias B. D. Wiggins, "You Are Here: Exploring Yoga and the Impact of Cultural Appropriation," featuring nisha ahuja, YouTube video, 25:24, June 17, 2014, www.youtube.com/watch?v=3OoBaDt9cvQ.

7 Sood, "Cultivating a Yogic Theology," 12.

8 Sood, 16.

9 Lakshmi Nair, "Even Spirit Has No Place to Call Home: Cultural Appropriation, Microaggressions, and Structural Racism in the Yoga Workplace," *Race and Yoga* 4, no. 1 (2019): 33.

10 Barkataki, "How to Decolonize Your Yoga Practice."

11 Prachi Patankar, "Ghosts of Yogas Past and Present," Jadaliyya, February 26, 2014, www.jadaliyya.com/Details/30281.

12 nisha ahuja, "You Are Here: Exploring Yoga and the Impacts of Cultural Appropriation," Soma Connection (blog), SOMA Integrative Wellness, September 7, 2018, www.somaintegrativewellness.com/you-are-here -exploring-yoga-and-the-impacts-of-cultural-appropriation.

13 Patankar, "Ghosts of Yogas Past and Present."

14 Ashwin Manthripragada, text message to author, November 30, 2020.

15 Eve Tuck and K. Wayne Yang, "Decolonization Is Not a Metaphor," *Decolonization: Indigeneity, Education & Society* 1, no. 1 (2012): 1.

16 Sheena Sood, "Towards a Critical Embodiment of Decolonizing Yoga," *Race and Yoga* 5, no. 1 (2020): 9.

17 Patty Adams, phone call with author, February 21, 2021.

18 Patrisse Cullors, "Abolition and Reparations: Histories of Resistance, Transformative Justice, and Accountability," *Harvard Law Review* 132, no. 6 (April 2019): 1686.

19 Susanna Barkataki, *Embrace Yoga's Roots: Courageous Ways to Deepen Your Yoga Practice* (Orlando, FL: Ignite Yoga and Wellness Institute, 2020), 237.

20 Molly Kitchen, email message to author, May 12, 2021.

21 Barkataki, "How to Decolonize Your Yoga Practice."

Liberatory Models of Yoga and Buddhism

1 Larry Yang, *Awakening Together: The Spiritual Practice of Inclusivity and Community* (Somerville, MA: Wisdom Publications, 2017), 69.

2 "EBMC Policies and Practices of Inclusion," Teacher Web: East Bay Meditation Center Teacher Sangha Resources, accessed May 10, 2021, https://teacherweb.eastbaymeditation.org/ebmc-policies-and-practices -of-inclusion.

3   Larry Yang, "Democracy Is Good for Sanghas," *Lion's Roar,* August 8, 2016, www.lionsroar.com/democracy-is-good-for-sanghas.

4   adrienne maree brown, *Emergent Strategy: Shaping Change, Changing Worlds* (Chico, CA: AK Press, 2017).

5   Krista Tippett, "Ruby Sales: Where Does It Hurt?," January 16, 2020, in *On Being,* podcast, MP3 audio, 52:09, https://onbeing.org/programs/ruby-sales-where-does-it-hurt.

6   Lisa Flynn and Bethany Butzer, "What We Can Learn from the Encinitas School Yoga Lawsuit: New Study Summary," Yoga 4 Classrooms blog, September 17, 2017, www.yoga4classrooms.com/yoga-4-classrooms-blog/what-we-can-learn-from-the-encinitas-school-yoga-lawsuit-new-study-summary.

7   Lindsay Kyte, "Where Everyone Can Thrive," *Lion's Roar,* July 1, 2018, www.lionsroar.com/where-everyone-can-thrive.

8   Kyte, "Where Everyone Can Thrive."

9   A reference to disability justice writer Eli Claire and the wisdom he shares in *Brilliant Imperfection: Grappling with Cure* (Durham, NC: Duke University Press, 2017).

Teaching Queer and Trans Yoga

1   "Murders of Transgender People in 2020 Surpasses Total for Last Year in Just Seven Months," National Center for Transgender Equality, August 7, 2020, https://transequality.org/blog/murders-of-transgender-people-in-2020-surpasses-total-for-last-year-in-just-seven-months.

2   Travis Alabanza, "Healing from Trauma as a Person of Colour: 3 Things I've Learnt as a Queer Black Boy," Black Girl Dangerous, April 21, 2015, www.blackgirldangerous.org/2015/04/healing-from-trauma-as-a-person-of-colour-3-things-ive-learnt-as-a-queer-black-boy.

3   Larry Yang, "Now More Than Ever," The Huffington Post, https://www.huffpost.com/entry/now-more-than-ever_b_1115434, December 1, 2011.

4   Alabanza, "Healing from Trauma as a Person of Colour."

5   Danny Arguetty, *Nourishing the Teacher: Inquiries, Contemplations, and Insights on the Path of Yoga,* 2nd ed. (San Diego: Nourish Your Light, 2009), 128.

6   John Lavitt, "Addiction Is a Response to Childhood Suffering: In Depth with Gabor Maté," The Fix, January 6, 2016, www.thefix.com/gabor-maté-addiction-holocaust-disease-trauma-recovery.

7   Grace Medley et al., *Sexual Orientation and Estimates of Adult Substance Use and Mental Health: Results from the 2015 National Survey on Drug Use and Health* (Rockville, MD: Substance Abuse and Mental Health Services Administration, October 2016), www.samhsa.gov/data/sites/default/files /NSDUH-SexualOrientation 2015/NSDUH-SexualOrientation-2015 /NSDUH-SexualOrientation-2015.htm.

8   Human Rights Campaign, *Preventing Substance Abuse Among LGBT Teens,* accessed December 9, 2020, www.hrc.org/resources/preventing-substance -abuse-among-lgbtq-teens.

9   Substance Abuse and Mental Health Services Administration, *A Provider's Introduction to Substance Abuse Treatment for Lesbian, Gay, Bisexual, and Transgender Individuals,* August 2012, https://store.samhsa.gov /product/A-Provider-s-Introduction-to-Substance-Abuse-Treatment -for-Lesbian-Gay-Bisexual-and-Transgender-Individuals/SMA12-4104.

10 New York University, "Lesbian, Gay, and Bisexual Older Adults at Higher Risk for Substance Use," June 2, 2020, www.nyu.edu/about/news -publications/news/2020/june/LGB-older-adults-substance-use.html.

11 Lavitt, "Addiction Is a Response to Childhood Suffering."

12 Becky Thompson, *Survivors on the Yoga Mat* (Berkeley, CA: North Atlantic Books, 2014), 167.

13 Lauren Paulk, "Sexual Assault in the LGBT Community," National Center for Lesbian Rights, April 30, 2014, www.nclrights.org/sexual-assault-in -the-lgbt-community.

Injustice Produces Trauma; Healing Creates Conditions for Justice

1   David Emerson, *Overcoming Trauma through Yoga: Reclaiming Your Body* (Berkeley, CA: North Atlantic Books, 2011), 35.

2   Tara Brach, "The Power of Radical Acceptance: Healing Trauma through the Integration of Buddhist Meditation and Psychotherapy," TaraBrach.com, accessed September 5, 2021, www.tarabrach.com /articles-interviews/trauma.

3   Tessa Hicks Peterson, *Student Development and Social Justice: Critical Learning, Radical Healing, and Community Engagement* (Cham, Switzerland: Palgrave McMillan, 2018), 92.

4   Anodea Judith, *Wheels of Life: The Classic Guide to the Chakra System* (Woodbury, MN: Llewellyn Worldwide, 1987), 4.

5   Lavitt, "Addiction Is a Response to Childhood Suffering."

6   Brach, "The Power of Radical Acceptance."

7   David A. Treleavan, *Trauma-Sensitive Mindfulness: Practices for Safe and Transformative Healing* (New York: W. W. Norton, 2018), 55.

8   Salzberg, *Lovingkindness,* 101.

9   Konda Mason, "Nonviolent Activism," in *Will Yoga and Meditation Really Change My Life?* ed. Stephen Cope (North Adams, MA: Storey Publishing, 2003), 113.

10   Hicks Peterson, *Student Development and Social Justice,* 79–80.

11   Jacoby Ballard and Karishma Kripalani, "Queering Yoga: An Ethic of Social Justice," in *Yoga, the Body, and Embodied Social Change: An Intersectional Feminist Analysis,* ed. Beth Berila, Melanie Klein, and Chelsea Jackson Roberts (Lanham, MD: Lexington Books, 2016), 304.

12   Danielle Sered, *Until We Reckon: Violence, Mass Incarceration, and a Road to Repair* (New York: The New Press, 2019), 231.

13   Hicks Peterson, *Student Development and Social Justice,* 112.

14   Hicks Peterson, 95.

15   Elisabeth Kübler-Ross, *Death: The Final Stage of Growth* (New York: Scribner, 1997), 96.

16   Desmond Tutu and Mpho Tutu, *The Book of Forgiving: The Fourfold Path for Healing Ourselves and Our World* (New York: HarperCollins, 2014), 24.

17   Krista Tippett, "Patrisse Cullors + Robert Ross: The Spiritual Work of Black Lives Matter," February 18, 2016, in *On Being,* podcast, MP3 audio, 51:49, https://onbeing.org/programs/patrisse-cullors-and-robert-ross-the-spiritual-work-of-black-lives-matter-may2017.

18   Zenju Earthlyn Manuel, *The Way of Tenderness: Awakening through Race, Sexuality, and Gender* (Somerville, MA: Wisdom Publications, 2015), 81.

19   Hicks Peterson, *Student Development and Social Justice,* 78.

20   Thompson, *Survivors on the Yoga Mat,* 183.

21   Loretta J. Ross, "Speaking Up without Tearing Down," *Learning for Justice,* Spring 2019, www.learningforjustice.org/magazine/spring-2019.

22   adrienne maree brown, "Learning and Untangling," adrienne maree brown (blog), August 1, 2020, http://adriennemareebrown.net/tag/call-out-culture/.

23   Alicia Garza, "Opening Ceremony Keynote," Allied Media Conference, June 16, 2017, https://alliedmedia.org/news/alicia-garza-speaks-building-power-amc2017-opening-ceremony.

24   Loretta Ross, "I'm a Black Feminist. I Think Call-Out Culture Is Toxic," *New York Times,* August 17, 2019, www.nytimes.com/2019/08/17/opinion /sunday/cancel-culture-call-out.html.

25   Maisha Z. Johnson, "6 Signs Your Call Out Is about Ego and Not Accountability," The Body Is Not an Apology (blog), May 22, 2019, https:// thebodyisnotanapology.com/magazine/6-signs-your-call-out-isnt -actually-about-accountability/.

26   adrienne maree brown, "Unthinkable Thoughts: Call Out Culture in the Age of COVID-19," adrienne maree brown (blog), July 17, 2020, http:// adriennemareebrown.net/2020/07/17/unthinkable-thoughts-call-out -culture-in-the-age-of-covid-19.

27   Garza, "Opening Ceremony Keynote."

28   Garza.

29   Haga, *Healing Resistance,* 107.

30   Manuel, *The Way of Tenderness,* 103.

31   Tutu and Tutu, *The Book of Forgiving,* 217.

32   Gregory Boyle, *Tattoos on the Heart: The Power of Boundless Compassion* (New York: Free Press, 2010), 177.

33   Angela Y. Davis, *Freedom Is a Constant Struggle: Ferguson, Palestine, and the Foundations of a Movement* (Chicago: Haymarket Books, 2016), 145.

34   Hala Khouri, "Conscious Activism," guest lecture in "Healing Ourselves in Healing Our Communities" course, Pitzer College, April 6, 2010, Claremont, CA, quoted in Hicks Peterson, *Student Development and Social Justice,* 68.

35   Tutu and Tutu, *The Book of Forgiving,* 97.

36   Thompson, *Survivors on the Yoga Mat,* 119.

37   Thompson, 199.

38   Hilda Gutiérrez Baldoquín, "Don't Waste Time," in *Dharma, Color, and Culture: New Voices in Western Buddhism,* ed. Hilda Gutiérrez Baldoquín (Berkeley, CA: Parallax Press, 2004), 182.

39   Alice Walker, "Edwidge Danticat, the Quiet Stream," Alice Walker: The Official Website, 2010, https://alicewalkersgarden.com/2010/01/edwidge -danticat-the-quiet-stream.

Conclusion: A Path from Here

1   Sebene Selassie, *You Belong: A Call for Connection* (New York: HarperOne, 2020), 202.

2   Bhagavad Gita 2:47 (trans. Stephen Mitchell).

3   Caitriona Reed, "Five Practices," Five Changes, accessed May 24, 2021, www.fivechanges.com/five-precepts.

4   Frances Lee, "Why I've Started to Fear My Fellow Social Justice Activists," *YES!,* October 13, 2017, www.yesmagazine.org/democracy/2017/10/13/why-ive-started-to-fear-my-fellow-social-justice-activists.

5   brown, "Unthinkable Thoughts."

6   Ngọc Loan Trần, "Calling IN: A Less Disposable Way of Holding Each Other Accountable," Black Girl Dangerous, December 18, 2013, www.bgdblog.org/2013/12/calling-less-disposable-way-holding-accountable.

7   Ross, "I'm a Black Feminist."

8   Ross, "Speaking Up without Tearing Down."

Appendix B: Pranayama Practices

1   Max Strom, "Breathe to Heal," TedxCapeMay, December 7, 2015, www.youtube.com/watch?v=4Lb5L-VEm34.

2   Brooke Donald, "Breathing Exercises Help Veterans Find Peace after War, Stanford Scholar Says," *Stanford Report,* May 22, 2013, https://news.stanford.edu/news/2013/may/veterans-breathing-study-052213.html.

3   Lindsay Tucker, "The Good Fight: How Yoga Is Being Used in the Military," *Yoga Journal,* September 27, 2018, www.yogajournal.com/lifestyle/how-yoga-is-being-used-within-the-military.

4   Sundar Balasubramanian, "The Science of Yogic Breathing," TEDx Charleston, YouTube video, 10:40, May 26, 2015, www.youtube.com/watch?v=aIfwbEvXtwo.

About the Author

JACOBY BALLARD (he/they) is a social justice educator and yoga teacher in Salt Lake City, Utah. He leads workshops and trainings around the country on diversity, equity, and inclusion and has consulted for Yoga Alliance, Lululemon, and Insight Meditation Society, among other organizations. As a yoga teacher with over two decades of experience, he leads weekly classes, workshops, and retreats and teaches in yoga teacher trainings around the country. Since 2006, Jacoby has taught Queer and Trans Yoga as a weekly class, a workshop, and a yoga retreat for LGBTQ communities, for which he received *Yoga Journal*'s Good Karma Award in 2016. In 2008, Jacoby founded Third Root Community Health Center in Brooklyn, New York, a worker-owned cooperative wellness center operating at the intersection of healing and social justice. Jacoby currently leads the Resonance Yoga Mentorship Program for yoga teachers to fill in gaps left out of many yoga teacher trainings, to work intimately with mentees, and help them find their gifts, niche, and calling. Jacoby has taught in gyms, schools, offices, universities, conferences, a cancer center, a recovery center, a homeless shelter, a maximum security prison, and yoga studios. Jacoby's teaching style is challenging and deep, playful and profound. Find Jacoby at jacobyballard.net, on Facebook, or on Instagram.

About North Atlantic Books